*Where
to Live
for Your
Health*

Where to Live for Your Health

Norman and
Madelyn Carlisle

Harcourt Brace Jovanovich
New York and London

Requests for permission to make copies of
any part of the work should be mailed to:
Permissions, Harcourt Brace Jovanovich, Inc.
757 Third Avenue, New York, N.Y. 10017

Printed in the United States of America

Library of Congress Cataloging in Publication Data

Carlisle, Norman V   1910–
Where to live for your health.

1. Climatology, Medical.   2.   Climatology,
Medical—United States.   3.   United States—Climate.
I. Carlisle, Madelyn, joint author.   II.   Title.
RA793.C29   613'.11'0973   79-2760
ISBN 0-15-196061-5

Set in Linotype Caledonia

First edition

B C D E

Contents

2085712

Foreword

As writers and reporters for national magazines we have done a lot of traveling and called many places home. Living in cities and in the country, in the desert and on mountains and beaches, in the North, South, East, and West, we've had an opportunity to experience all kinds of climates. As we added to the list of places where we had sojourned we became increasingly conscious of the impact weather and climate had on the way we felt, physically and mentally.

Wherever we lived and traveled we talked to people. One of the first things we asked almost everybody was, "Did you move here from somewhere else?" And then, of course, followed all the related questions: "Why did you move?" "How long have you been here?" "Do you like it?" "Do you feel any different?"

We found that there's been a change in the reasons people give for moving. Two or three decades ago it seemed the adventurous, or perhaps the economic, thing to do. Today more Americans move because they are looking for "a better place to live."

After questioning people's motivations for leaving one place and going to live in another, pollster Lou Harris pronounced, "Most Americans today don't want more *quantity* of anything; they want more *quality*." The reason most frequently given for moving was "to find a better quality of life."

In anyone's thoughts about a better life, health looms as a paramount factor. Today when we ask people why they moved, the answers are likely to run along these lines: "We just had to get away from the smog" . . . "I didn't want to live with all that noise and dirt" . . . "I couldn't stand the humidity" . . . "We wanted a more healthful place to raise our kids" . . . "Well, I have a heart condition and I'd like to live as long as I can" . . . "I felt it would help my arthritis" . . . "My sinuses couldn't take it anymore."

Many of the people we talked to were retirees. But we found young people just out of college—even just out of high school—who were thinking in terms of finding more healthful places to live. Even people in perfectly good health express the hope that any change they make will bring them a still more healthful existence, with, perhaps, cleaner air, less humidity, more sunshine, and not so much of a struggle with excessive cold or heat or other troublesome elements in the weather.

What had been simply a personal interest for a number of years gradually developed into something a great deal more. It became a different kind of journey—an exploration into the world of human biometeorology, the science which, drawing its practitioners from many disciplines, studies the influences of weather, climate, and other environmental factors on people. Biometeorologists include meteorologists, climatologists, ecologists, geographers, archaeologists, biologists, chemists, psychologists, and physicians from many medical specialties. To them we owe most of the contents of this book.

If you're hoping that through our research and reportorial efforts we've found some magical Shangri-La that will guarantee you good health and long life and that we're going to tell you where it is, we're sorry to disappoint you. There is no place that's best for everybody. As Roger Williams, the noted biochemist of the University of Texas, said, "There's nobody else like you." Individual reactions to everything—weather, climate, and environment included—vary so widely that what may be right for one person may be wrong for another. However, there certainly are some absolutes, and there are guidelines you can use.

If you are one of those thinking about setting out on a quest for a better place to live, we hope that this book will make your life a happier and healthier one by . . .

- giving you a better understanding of just what weather is doing for you and to you;
- showing you how to cope with some of the dangers of environmental hazards, such as polluted air and contaminated drinking water;
- introducing you to a little-known factor in the air that may have a profound effect on your well-being wherever you live;
- giving you an understanding of how the weather affects various chronic illnesses—arthritis, sinusitis, bronchitis, asthma, allergies, heart conditions;
- telling you how to find a climate that's better for you.

NORMAN AND MADELYN CARLISLE

New Mexico
August 1979

*Where
to Live
for Your
Health*

1

Weather

Weather—the marvelous, exciting, variable combination of meteorological factors—is the cutting edge of climate. The pressure of the air, the amount of moisture it holds, its temperature, and the kinds and amounts of electrified particles in it act upon us every minute of our lives. In different combinations, modified by season, latitude, altitude, relationship to mountains or bodies of water, movements of air masses, storms, winds, sunlight, and pollutants in the air, these weather phenomena exert profound influences on our well-being.

Biometeorologists who have made extensive studies of people's responses to weather report an astonishing range of effects on human health. The catalog of ills that can be weather-caused includes the following:

fatigue	irritability
headache	nervousness
migraine	anxiety
rheumatic pain	depression
bone fracture pain	vomiting
impaired concentration	insomnia
forgetfulness	moist palms
confusion	excessive sweating
tendency to make mistakes	hot flushes
exhaustion	convulsive tics

chills

dislike of work

inability to work

lack of appetite

diarrhea

frequent urination

head pressure

hearing disturbances

smell disturbances

taste disturbances

vision disturbances

skin sensitivity

scar pain

vertigo

faintness

heart palpitations

respiratory problems

breathlessness

general discomfort

It's an appalling list of ailments, and chances are that you have suffered from several of them without ever realizing that the weather was the culprit. Every one of us, no matter what our age, sex, or state of health, is affected in some way by what the weather is doing.

What the Weather Does to You

You may well be wondering how the weather can have such an impact on you in this age of air-conditioned and evenly heated comfort, when most of us spend much of our time indoors anyway. While a majority of the people we've talked to about weather and its effects have agreed that they are usually at the mercy of the weather, we've also run into some skeptics.

"No, the weather doesn't bother me. I'm not out in it for more than an hour a day," was a comment we heard many times.

No matter if you *never* go outside, certain factors in the weather are inescapable. Even a person who is outside only for an hour a day, according to Dr. Solco Tromp, head of the Biometeorological Research Centre in the Netherlands, is affected: "If a subject remains out of doors for an hour, and probably even less, he will sustain a physiological imprint for twelve hours or more that is characteristic of the meteorological conditions of that particular day, even if he spends the remainder of the day in an air-conditioned environment with a constant climate."

In other words, if you go outdoors for just *one hour,* your body will respond to that exposure for the next twelve hours.

How can the weather do that? What happens is that all of the body's organs and systems undergo changes that correspond to factors in the weather.

The *endocrine glands* constitute the bodily mechanism most profoundly and directly affected. They serve to bring about many of the other bodily responses to meteorological activities through the hormones they emit. The hormones produced in greater or lesser profusion by glands responding to atmospheric conditions regulate many of the body's vital functions.

Blood is affected in many ways. The amount of blood increases or decreases, with variations in the quantity of blood cells and blood serum. Speeding up or slowing down the time required for blood clotting often accounts for hemorrhaging of postoperative patients under certain weather conditions. The weather also brings about marked changes in blood constituents, including calcium, magnesium, phosphate, and iodine.

The *heart* beats faster or slower, producing changes in blood pressure.

Breathing rate responds to some weather conditions, with your capacity to take in air being reduced as much as 30 percent under some conditions. Such a slowdown obviously reduces the amount of oxygen in the blood.

The *cellular water content* changes, causing some parts of the body to swell.

Muscles undergo metabolic changes that affect their strength and the speed with which they respond to nerve impulses. You can actually be stronger on some days than on others, thanks to the weather.

In view of all the physiological changes your body undergoes in response to the weather, it is little wonder that your psychological state reflects them. We are all aware that our spirits can sag when skies remain cloudy day after day and that they can soar when we awaken to a fresh, sunny morning. But there are many other, not so obvious, effects exerted by the weather on your mental state.

Are you needlessly cross with your best friend, your children, or your spouse? The weather may be at the bottom of your irritability. The weather on a given day can even limit your mental efficiency, make you inept and incapable of carrying out your work.

Are You Weather-Sensitive?

These changes are something we all experience, in some degree. One of the major discoveries of the biometeorologists is that some of us are much more affected than others. One out of three persons, they say, is *meteorotropic*—or, in layman's language, "weather-sensitive." If you are weather-sensitive you respond with greater intensity to some or all of the weather phenomena that exert influences on the human body.

Weather-sensitive people are affected by all the complaints on the list but, in each instance, to a greater extent. For example, fatigue holds first place on the weather-induced ailments list of both weather-sensitive and non-weather-sensitive persons. Twenty-one percent of non–weather sensitives suffer this discomfort, compared to 57 percent of weather-sensitive people. Fourteen percent of the non–weather sensitives blame their irritability on the weather at times; for the weather sensitives the percentage is 48.

Dislike of work? Among non–weather sensitives, 16 percent are aware of the fact that, under certain weather conditions, they just don't want to work, whereas 45 percent of weather-sensitive people say they "often" have to drag themselves to their jobs.

"Weather sensitivity might almost be described as an allergy to the weather," said one medical researcher.

You can be weather-sensitive at some time in your life and not in another. Children and adolescents are the least susceptible, with only 24 percent in the thirteen-to-twenty-six age group affected. The rate climbs to 33 percent for the twenty-to-fifty-year-olds. The most afflicted, for reasons not yet known, are those between fifty and sixty. After the age of sixty the figure drops back down to 24 percent.

Sex is also a factor in the incidence of weather sensitivity. There are about twice as many female victims as there are male sufferers. Biometeorologists believe this is because females do not produce stress hormones in the quantities that males do.

The Doctor, the Patient, and the Weather

Biometeorology has not reached the point where your doctor will diagnose your weather ills or give you a prescription for a climate where you might do better. However, there is greater interest in biometeorology than ever before. An editorial in the *Journal of the American Medical Association* told its physician readers: "There is currently considerable discussion concerning environmental pollution. However, climate and weather, important environmental factors that influence the health of the people of America *to an even greater extent* [our italics], receive relatively little attention as health problems. Although pollution may be controlled, climate and weather cannot be, and therefore man cannot escape entirely the stresses of weather and climate. Man must learn to maintain the best possible health in spite of his climate and weather. It should be the duty of the medical profession to aid in this learning."

Most doctors accept the fact that weather is an important medical consideration. When Dr. Sidney Licht, a Yale professor of medicine, set out to compile a textbook in the field of biometeorology, he conducted a survey of Board Certified internists in all fifty states.

Among other questions Dr. Licht asked was this one: "Do you believe that there is any significant relationship between the symptoms of disease and weather?" Only 2 percent saw no relationship; 6 percent were on the fence; and 92 percent of the respondents answered "yes."

It is surprising that there are any doctors who can discount the influences of weather on human health in view of the four-volume work *The Patient and the Weather* by Dr. William Petersen. This Chicago doctor started his career as a professor of histology at the University of Illinois School of Medicine. He wasn't thinking about the weather when he undertook a research project in an area of medicine that both puzzled and fascinated him. He had observed that there were many differences in patients that seemed to contradict standard medical statements about "normal" functioning. What really was the "normal" range for pulse rate? The "normal" range for sugar content of the blood?

With an associate, Petersen set up a program that called for making all kinds of tests on all kinds of people.

"We practically pulled them in off the street," he reported later. "What did it do for us? Well, we finished up a couple of years later with a pile of records and a rather distressing conclusion. Everyone we tested was different. So-called normal was meaningless."

Petersen decided that instead of testing so many people, he should make much more intensive studies of just a few patients over a long period of time. He selected six patients for his study and tested them daily for twelve different physical reactions. After eighteen months of this daily checking, he and his associates tabulated their results. They confirmed the earlier findings that there was no "normal." Each patient showed distinctive readings.

But the tabulations showed something else—something that startled the researchers. Allowing for the individual differences, all the patients showed the same *pattern* of variations from day to day. When one registered high blood sugar, so did the others. When oxygen in the blood of one was down, it was down in all.

"We sat down and scratched our heads," Petersen commented. "Why was this happening? We couldn't figure it out. A hundred and one explanations came to our minds but none of them satisfied us. What could be the common denominator? The only one we could think of was the weather.

"We didn't even take the possibility seriously, but as a gesture—and a half-hearted one at that—we charted the weather for the period and compared it with our medical records. No one could have been more surprised than I was to find that daily weather changes and daily body changes were going along together."

Later, in *The Patient and the Weather,* Dr. Petersen reported thousands of observations on how hundreds of patients responded to weather influences. No one before or since has made so many detailed studies on so many patients over such a long period of time. Today, more than forty years later, it still stands as the monumental work in the field of biometeorology.

The science is no longer dependent upon the observations of such dedicated iconoclasts as Dr. Petersen. For one thing, researchers have a lot more detailed weather-climate-environment information to draw on. Thousands of ground observation stations, weather balloons, and satellites in space are daily pouring out a vast amount of data for computers to digest and analyze. For the first time, we have a series of readings that can be related to human responses.

Scientists also have the use of a wonderful new research tool—the climate chamber: a room or suite of rooms in which all the "weather" factors can be varied at will. The climate chamber is as important to the advance of biometeorology as the microscope has been to the advance of medicine in general.

Using the climate chamber, researchers have made major contributions to biometeorological knowledge. Their findings have, as one physician pointed out to us, "made biometeorology a science we can really begin to put to practical use."

As more Americans question their doctors about places that might be better for their health, more and more physicians are getting a chance to do just that.

A Phoenix rheumatologist told us, "I have at least a hundred patients who have moved here from someplace else. In witnessing the effects the change of climate has had on these newcomers, I've become a student of biometeorology myself."

2

Up and Down with the Barometer

Do you have days when you feel depressed, irritated by trifles, absentminded, quick to argue? When you spill things, or drop them, or lose them, or find your fingers are all thumbs? When you can't seem to think straight? When you somehow just don't feel up to par? When any chronic ills you have are at their worst? Your reactions may be traceable to the fact that, even though the sky is clear and the breezes gentle, somewhere off there, maybe still a couple of days away, a large air mass is moving in your direction. And already, where you are, the barometer is falling.

In the standard mercurial barometer, the air pushes down on the open end of a U-shaped tube containing mercury. At sea level, under standard conditions, the atmosphere balances the column of mercury at 29.92 inches. In other words, normal barometric pressure is 29.92. When we say the barometer is "falling," we really mean the column of mercury is going down. This means that air pressure has lessened. If the air pressure goes up, or increases, the column of mercury rises.

A barometer is extremely sensitive to changes in air pressure—

and so are you. Your body, a sensitive weather instrument itself, cannot help but be affected by the ups and downs of atmospheric pressure. Changes in atmospheric pressure can do far more than cause you mental and physical distress. By exacerbating any ailments with which you're already saddled, they can inflict upon you not only pain and discomfort, but sometimes even threats to your life.

The North American continent is constantly being crossed, from west to east, by large air masses—or storms, as the meteorologists call them. When a high-pressure air mass, which is warm, meets a low-pressure air mass, which is cold, the interface between them is called a "front," and this is where weather changes begin to occur.

Many of the weather upheavals created by these clashing air masses move across what meteorologists term the "U.S. Storm Belt." Their paths may vary, but almost all of them pass over New England before they journey out across the Atlantic to Europe. However, by the time these storm movements cross New England, they have lost a lot of their vigor. So, though storms may be more frequent in the northeastern states, they are not, on the average, as violent as those that batter the great central plains.

"North America is unique in that its population is subject to greater meteorological demands than any other densely inhabited region in the world," said Dr. William Petersen. He saw storms as playing the role of villain in many diseases of the body. Many other researchers attribute an awesome catalog of mental and emotional ills to the roller-coaster ups and downs of the weather.

Many atmospheric changes accompany storm movements. Pressure, humidity, temperature, and the electrical properties of the atmosphere all fluctuate. Not only do storms bother all of us to some degree, and weather-sensitive people in particular, while they're where we are; but they affect us before they've come and after they've gone. Long before you can see the effects of a change in weather, it's doing something to the ocean of air in which you live. As it reaches the place where you are, it hits you with other effects. And as it passes it leaves you physiologically reeling in an attempt to recover your equilibrium.

Heralds of Changing Weather

Long before biometeorology—or even meteorology—became a science, it had been observed that the behavior of animals sometimes foretells the coming of a storm. Horses rear and bolt for no apparent reason. "Another runaway—must be going to rain," was a common remark. Hogs and other farm animals can become belligerent, attacking one another without provocation. Normally friendly dogs act snappish and restless. Dr. Clarence Mills once kept a record and found that the number of stray dogs picked up by dogcatchers increased on days when a storm was brewing. "For safety's sake," he advised, "confine your petting of strange canines to days when barometric pressure is rising."

Fishermen have a lot of explanations as to why fish do or do not bite on a particular day or when the weather is behaving one way or another, but biometeorologists theorize that it is atmospheric pressure that influences them most strongly. The fish are triggered into activity—in this case, bait snatching—when there is a change in the barometer. So next time you have a catch that's worth bragging about, check what the barometer's been doing and let it be your guide as to when to go and try your luck again.

The fact that people respond as do other creatures to forthcoming storms was thought to be just a bit of folklore until an American teacher brought it into the realm of modern science. At the time—the late 1890s—Edwin Dexter was a professor of education and psychology at the University of Illinois. One day when classroom discipline was under discussion a student asked him, "Have you ever noticed that on days when the weather is bad children are harder to manage?"

Of course he'd noticed that, Dexter glibly replied, and the

reason was obvious. A rainy day kept children indoors and deprived them of normal outlets for their energy. Then, too, in bad weather, the windows were closed and the classrooms stuffy.

Dexter might well have forgotten all about the discussion but for the fact that the next day the students brought up the subject again. Some of them had already had teaching experience and they expressed doubt that the professor's explanation was adequate. They had noted that pupils were sometimes noticeably restless on clear days as well. How did Dexter account for that?

When he couldn't explain it, Dexter set out to do some research. He soon found that almost nothing on the subject existed in print. By this time he was hooked. When his summer vacation started he set out on a quest that was going to take him years.

In the New York Police Department files he pored over musty records from half a century back to find out if there was an increase in crime under certain weather conditions. In New York and other cities he went over the records of hospital admissions. Was there a connection between weather and illness, particularly mental illness? He talked to people, interviewing literally thousands of doctors, lawyers, psychologists, teachers, prison wardens, police officials, and meteorologists.

Eventually Dexter accumulated such a vast store of data that he could base his conclusions on more than a million individual cases of sickness, misconduct, emotional disturbance, and death. He made many observations about the influences of temperature and humidity, but his most important discovery was the answer to the original question that had prompted his research. The mysterious factor that made children restless was not rain that was actually falling, but rain that was *going* to fall. The children were reacting, Dexter concluded, to the combination of meteorological factors involved in oncoming storms.

The researches of present-day biometeorologists confirm Dexter's findings. They have turned up a stunning array of evidence that storms, particularly for those who live in the storm belt, cause many mental and emotional woes.

The Phases of a Storm

The approach, passage, and aftermath of the movement of large air masses—some may be 1,000 miles across—produce a number of meteorological effects, which can be seen on the accompanying diagram. It divides a storm into six phases. Phase 1, at the far right, is the first that hits you. As the storm moves you are successively assailed by phases 2, 3, and so on. Phases 3, 4, and 5 are the most uncomfortable ones.

Although humidity and temperature play a role in creating physiological reactions, the most distressing phenomenon associated with storms is the drop in barometric pressure. Changes in pressure occur because the atmosphere pushes down with varying weight as masses of cold or warm air move about above us. (High-pressure air masses weigh more than the air surrounding them; low-pressure masses weigh less.)

The barometer falls as any front approaches—either warm or cold. It rises again after a storm has passed. If a warm front is approaching, the barometer falls steadily, then rises and falls erratically as the storm front passes. A cold front heralds its approach by a slow drop at first, then a rapid one as the front gets close. Some storm conditions cause wild movement of the barometer, with many ups and downs. They may occur within a few hours or be spread out over days.

Are You a Storm Victim?

Biometeorologists don't know exactly how storm phases affect the human body, but they do know that the effects are many. First of all, when the barometer fluctuates, bodily tissues alternately swell and shrink, creating painful symptoms in many people. When the pressure drops, it is believed that the intestinal tract gives up water, which goes into other parts of the body, causing them to enlarge. When the pressure rises, the reverse process occurs. The swelling resulting from the influx of water may be minute in some people but very pronounced in others.

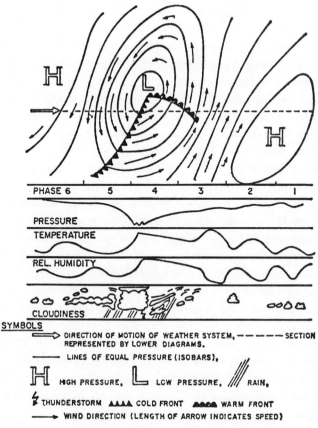

Schematic representation of the six phases of a storm. Each phase
in this diagram spans twenty-four hours; in reality the phases may
be shorter or longer. (International Society of Biometeorologists)

In the case of one patient who suffered rheumatic pains before
a storm, it was found that her legs, which continued to swell for
the duration of the barometer's slide, sometimes actually increased an inch in girth.

Another possible explanation for why a drop in barometric
pressure causes discomfort may be that normal barometric pressure tends to hold joints in place and to keep capillaries at
normal diameter. A drop in pressure could, therefore, cause joints

to loosen, resulting in pain for the arthritic, and capillaries to dilate, creating difficulties for some allergics.

Several other events take place in a storm-wracked body. One of the most marked physiological effects is a change in the oxygen supply to various body organs.

"When we examine the blood pressure of a perfectly normal individual living in the storm tracks we find that the level is changing from day to day," says Dr. Petersen. "This means that at certain times when the blood vessels are contracting not all the tissues are being well supplied with blood. There is at least a partial oxygen inadequacy. This will become particularly apparent in the cerebral blood vessels, the blood vessels of the heart, the kidneys, the skin and special sense organs. As a result these organs will be stimulated because of this oxygen hunger. In turn, substances are formed which dilate vessels all over the body. As they dilate, blood pressure falls."

This may not particularly harm the normal individual. Healthy persons often take the pummeling of the weather comfortably in stride and show no observable response. They might notice only changes in mood, feeling optimistic and energetic on one day and sluggish and depressed the next. However, clinical effects do show up in the case of people who have some organic problem. Vascular spasm and oxygen hunger may so stimulate an ailing organ that fatigue or actual injury results.

For example, when a cold front approaches, the body "tightens up," sugar is mobilized from the liver, blood pressure rises, muscle tone increases, metabolic rate climbs. As the storm passes, the body restores itself to its pre-storm condition: muscles relax and blood pressure falls. This is stressful, even for an absolutely healthy body, and if the body has any weaknesses it can have a hard time making these changes. If storms follow one another in quick succession, your body can be kept in a constant state of stress as it tries to adjust to overlapping conditions.

"The weather in turmoil can create a body in turmoil," Dr. Petersen once remarked in a conversation with the authors. He established a long list of human ailments that were traceable to cold fronts in particular. Dr. Petersen's list of ailments ranged through almost the entire spectrum of human afflictions—from gallbladder attacks, flare-ups of gastric ulcers, and migraine headaches to much more serious problems, such as hemorrhages and heart attacks.

Asthma sufferers, for example, have been found to be especially responsive to storm conditions. Many reports in the medical literature describe situations in which there are sudden rashes of asthma attacks.

Dr. John Peters, another Chicago physician, and one of the many medical people influenced by Dr. Petersen, kept extensive records of the weather's relationship to his patients' ailments. He often astonished colleagues who were less aware of weather influences by predicting that within twenty-four hours they would have to deal with an unusually large number of bronchial asthma cases. He based his always accurate medical forecasts on barometric readings.

"There's going to be a change in the weather. I feel it in my bones," has been a commonplace utterance, probably as long as man has suffered from rheumatic diseases. Doctors no longer have any doubts about the veracity of patients who insist they can foretell a storm by the increase in their aches and pains. Experiments carried out in the University of Pennsylvania's climate chamber under the direction of Dr. J. L. Hollander have also shown that many arthritis patients are responsive to barometric ups and downs. (See Chapter 14 for a full discussion.)

Pressure and Performance

Storm conditions prompt more than physical reactions. All of us—weather-sensitive and non-weather-sensitive alike—contend with the influence of fluctuations in atmospheric pressure on our mental and emotional states. Our moods, our ability to cope with daily tasks, even our outlook on life on a given day are all conditioned by the pressure of the air around us. Scientists have an explanation for the mental and psychological effects that accompany storms. They theorize that an increase in the water content of the blood vessels lessens the oxygen supply to the brain, just as it does to other body organs.

"A low barometer can make you uncomfortable," says Dr. Clarence Mills, the often-quoted University of Cincinnati researcher. "Adults tend to feel frustrated, quarrelsome, emotionally upset. Children become irritable." Depression, restlessness, insomnia, anxiety, and forgetfulness are just a few of the other symptoms Dr. Mills has traced to storms.

Studies in prisons show that prisoners are more unruly on low-pressure days. In a private school a record of demerits given to students for misbehavior followed exactly the pattern of pressure changes; low pressure brought a high number of demerits. Suicide rates also climb when the barometer is low.

"Inadequate oxidation in cells and tissues is an important explanation of psychiatric disorders. And this is weather-linked, biochemically measurable, and clinically obvious," reports Dr. Hans R. Reese, University of Wisconsin neuropsychiatrist.

Storm-related effects on people explain a puzzling increase in traffic accidents on days that seem to provide perfect driving conditions. The temperature can be moderate, the sky clear, the road dry, yet tailgating accidents and head-on collisions may occur in record-breaking numbers.

"It's as if a lot of drivers are half-asleep," was the remark of a state trooper patrolling the New York Thruway on a particularly disastrous day.

Researchers at Queens University in Kingston, Ontario, have established that these deadly clear-weather accident days are linked to bad weather that hasn't yet arrived. After analyzing statistics and relating them to weather phenomena, the Canadian biometeorologists determined that 75 percent of nonfatal accidents over a period of months on Ontario highways occurred when the barometer was falling, indicating an approaching storm. Even more of the fatal accidents—a chilling 81 percent—occurred on such days.

What happens to the drivers to make them accident-prone on

these days? Numerous studies like the Ontario one have provided the answer, but none more decisively than a test that wasn't intended as a biometeorological experiment at all.

The weather was far from the minds of the managers of an automobile safety show in Berlin when they set up facilities for checking the reaction times of visitors. The apparatus was simple. A person taking the test just pushed a button when a traffic light set up in a booth changed color. An automatic device registered the lag between the time the light changed and the time the visitor pushed the button.

As was expected, it was found that there was a lot of variation in people's reaction times. But, as the testing went on over a period of ten weeks, involving over 20,000 people, something quite unexpected turned up. On some days the group-average reaction times were definitely higher, while on other days they slowed down. Why? Biometeorologists who examined the data were able to come up with an explanation. The slow-reaction days were those when the city was the center of a low-pressure system. After the storm passed, reactions speeded up again.

Should You Flee the Storm Belt?

If you live in the storm belt, you may want to find out what storms are doing to *you*. Your vulnerability—or lack of it—to their various effects will probably become apparent if you keep a record of barometric pressure and your reactions to it. Winter is the ideal season to keep such records, since winter storms are more volatile and more frequent, move faster, and generally have worse effects on weather-sensitive people than do storms at other times of the year.

If you find out—or already know—that your body and psyche take a beating from the troubled atmosphere, what should you do? You might consider moving. This is good advice for anyone, regardless of age, but especially for older people and people who have chronic ills that are storm-affected. Dr. Petersen's advice should be considered seriously: "Get out of the storm belt!"

"I've become a different person," a former Boston engineer told us, "since I moved to Florida. I used to be a nervous wreck for days at a time, then I'd mysteriously—that is, it was mysterious to me at the time—feel strangely calm and in control of things. Tranquilizers helped, but I began to get worried about my dependency on them. Now I don't take any at all. Of course, I don't know that it was only the barometric ups and downs that were causing my trouble, but I know they played a big part in it. I kept careful enough records to show me that there was a distinct relationship."

Bearing Up under Barometric Pressure

If you're in no position to move, there isn't much you can do to control your reactions to storm conditions. But you may be able to minimize the impact of their psychological effects. You'd do well to heed one of Dr. Mills's prescriptions: "Proper appreciation of their [storms'] presence will take much of the stress and unpleasantness out of life in stormy regions. In my own family greater tolerance is exercised on those days when we know we can expect each other to be more restless and irritable. I have learned in my own work that some days are good only for routine jobs while on others difficult tasks are readily accomplished.

"If you are in business avoid your most difficult customer on falling-pressure days. His instinctive reaction is more likely to be curt and unfavorable. Call on him when fair weather and a rising barometer are standing by as your allies. Attack your most difficult problems on the mornings of rising-pressure days."

We know of a Minneapolis family rent with dissension. Quarrels erupted at the slightest provocation. The marriage seemed about to break up. The wife told us, "It hardly seemed reasonable to suppose the weather had anything to do with it, but my husband read an article in the newspaper about some biometeorologist who said that storms made some people restless, and he was impressed by it. My husband thought that maybe we'd find that our worst quarrels had something to do with storms. We started checking the barometer, and I found that storms certainly were a factor. It turned out that I was the culprit, because it was plain from our record that whenever the barometer was falling I became irritable and would easily fly off the handle over trifles.

"Of course, finding this out didn't end all our troubles, but knowing it certainly made things easier. For instance, by not talking about such troublesome subjects as money when the weather isn't on my side, I manage to keep from blowing my stack a lot of the time. And my husband has been a lot more considerate since he now realizes that sometimes I'm just reacting to the weather, something that is completely beyond my control."

Heed the impact of storm conditions on your own psychological and mental states and try to avoid tasks that call for intense concentration under weather conditions that slow your reactions and make you mentally sluggish. Don't blame yourself for making mistakes or for being absentminded. Avoid family discussions that might lead to arguments when the barometer is falling if you've recognized the fact that you or members of your family are prone to irritability when atmospheric pressure is low. Conversely, plan to do things that call for confidence, high spirits, and mental and physical efficiency on days when your reactions to what the weather is doing are in your favor.

No place is completely free of barometric ups and downs. Localized storms occur everywhere. However, you can escape the big air movements that cause the most trouble. Even northerners who like the cold and snow leave it behind to get away from the violent upheavals, the dramatic weather swings, the sheer stress of constantly having to adjust to changing conditions.

On the other hand, there are people who find it hard to adapt to more stable climates, a fact that accounts for many of the vague feelings of discontent often expressed to us by retirees to southern states. "Sure, the Gulf Coast is a great place to live," one told us, "but I miss the kind of weather we had in Indiana. I had more energy there."

Biometeorologists go along with that statement. They even agree that, for some people, changeable weather, even violent storminess, may be beneficial. As one biometeorologist said to us, "Some people have systems that just roll with the punches and they actually seem to enjoy, even to need, that kind of 'meteorological massage.'"

3

Should You Run Away from the Cold?

We have observed that people complain more about cold than about any other single aspect of the weather. Some people, of course, say they like cold, but it usually turns out that it isn't really the cold they like, but cold-weather sports and activities.

Man as a species had his beginnings in tropical regions; we still seem to function best when air temperatures are neither too hot nor too cold. Ask almost anyone what temperature he or she finds most comfortable and the answer is likely to be, "Oh, about seventy-five degrees." It is certainly no coincidence that medical researches reveal that man's cardiovascular system operates at its optimum and that the fewest deaths occur when the temperature is between 60 and 79 degrees Fahrenheit.

Few of us are so fortunate as to never have to cope with cold. Ever since our distant ancestors left their warm equatorial cradle and ventured into harsher climes, a large percentage of mankind has had to spend a large percentage of its time struggling to keep warm. Early man covered himself with animal skins and huddled, when he could, around his fires. Only the need for food drove him out into the cold, snow, and wind. Even today, points out Dr. Helmut Landsberg, former chief climatologist of the National Weather Service, "man has not developed a race that can naturally survive in cold regions. Only technology has enabled him to do so."

We might argue with him on that point. The Eskimos have done quite well for a long time with precious little technology to aid them. And one must remember Darwin's surprise upon finding that the natives of Tierra del Fuego went around stark naked, with the snow and sleet pelting their bodies, in temperatures ranging from 3° C. to 7° C. (roughly 37° F. to 45° F.), even sleeping on the cold, wet ground at night without covering.

Even today, in the modern technological age, people caught unprepared and unsheltered in the cold still suffer dire consequences and can even lose their lives. Almost none of us is physiologically equipped to survive without heat and shelter in the cold. In addition to the cold, there is also the wind-chill factor to contend with. In still air, the human body, if it is insulated enough, builds up a nice cushion of warm air between the skin and what is covering it. But the moving air of the wind can often carry away that protection.

You can tell how much wind speed influences temperature effects from the accompanying chart. For example, a 20-mph wind blowing when the temperature is 5° F. will make you feel as cold as you would be in a still-air temperature of −31° F.

The effect of any drop in temperature is greatly increased when it's accompanied by a wind. At a temperature of 30° F., with a 36-mph wind, a drop of three degrees will change people's opinions of the temperature from "very cold" to "bitter cold." At that same 30° F., with a wind of 6 mph blowing, it takes the *ten times* greater drop in temperature of thirty Fahrenheit degrees, from 30° F. down to zero, to make the response change from "very cold" to "bitter cold." (See the Wind Chill Equivalent Temperature graph.)

What Cold Does to Your Body

The Department of Energy has issued a pronouncement that thermostats should be set at 68° F. in the winter months, but

WIND-CHILL EQUIVALENT TEMPERATURE GRAPH

DRY BULB TEMPERATURE (°F)

WIND VELOCITY (MPH)	45	40	35	30	25	20	15	10	5	0	-5	-10	-15	-20	-25	-30	-35	-40	-45	
4	45	40	35	30	25	20	15	10	5	0	-5	-10	-15	-20	-25	-30	-35	-40	-45	4
5	43	37	32	27	22	16	11	6	0	-5	-10	-15	-21	-26	-31	-36	-42	-47	-52	5
10	34	28	22	16	10	3	-3	-9	-15	-22	-27	-34	-40	-46	-52	-58	-64	-71	-77	10
15	29	23	16	9	2	-5	-11	-18	-25	-31	-38	-45	-51	-58	-65	-72	-78	-85	-92	15
20	26	19	12	4	-3	-10	-17	-24	-31	-39	-46	-53	-60	-67	-74	-81	-88	-95	-103	20
25	23	16	8	1	-7	-15	-22	-29	-36	-44	-51	-59	-66	-74	-81	-88	-96	-103	-110	25
30	21	13	6	-2	-10	-18	-25	-33	-41	-49	-56	-64	-71	-79	-86	-93	-101	-109	-116	30
35	20	12	4	-4	-12	-20	-27	-35	-43	-52	-58	-67	-74	-82	-89	-97	-105	-113	-120	35
40	19	11	3	-5	-13	-21	-29	-37	-45	-53	-60	-69	-76	-84	-92	-100	-107	-115	-123	40
45	18	10	2	-6	-14	-22	-30	-38	-46	-54	-62	-70	-78	-85	-93	-102	-109	-117	-125	45

The shaded squares illustrate the fact that at a temperature of 20° F., with the wind blowing at 10 mph, the wind-chill equivalent temperature is 3° F. (National Climatic Center) many people insist they aren't comfortable unless the setting is at least 75. Others think they might settle for 72. However, for most Americans, anything less than that seems to induce shivers.

Are we a nation of softies? Middle Europeans don't mind indoor temperatures of 65 and the British vow that 60 is quite a good setting. Our reactions to cold, in other words, are to a large extent a matter of what we are used to. However, all of us—no matter what country we live in or what our ethnic background may be—share the same physiological mechanisms for responding to cold. We all have embedded in our skins a network of cold sensors, which are responsive to minute changes in temperature. When they feel a drop they relay a message to the thermoregulatory centers of the brain. The prompt response of these centers is to order a step-up in metabolism, commanding the body to produce more heat. The thyroid and other glands that control metabolism are helped along by muscular responses. One of them is shivering, a kind of forced exercise of large numbers of muscles, which, by their movement, produce heat.

Your age has a lot to do with how much you "feel the cold" and how your body responds to it. Since your circulation slows down somewhat as you get older, your system delivers less blood to the skin. Therefore your skin temperature may be lower to begin with, so that when you enter a cold room or step out into the outdoor cold, you can become instantly chilled.

Body build is also a factor. Fat people suffer more from heat, but less from cold, than thin people do. However, army tests show that while men of heavier weight and larger build generally feel more comfortable in cold situations than men of smaller build, the small, leaner ones who suffer the most when they're actually out in the cold bounce back faster and experience fewer ill effects after they get back in where it's warm.

Physically fit individuals, because they have better-functioning cardiovascular systems and better blood flow to their extremities, adapt to cold much better than those who are not in good shape. Malnourished people are extremely sensitive to cold. Subjected to cold stress, they are likely to fall victim to infection because they don't have the bodily reserves that fight off invading organisms.

Do you suffer from cold feet? A standard explanation is "poor circulation," but your frigid toes don't necessarily mean there's something wrong with your circulation. Quite the contrary; they may be a good indication that there's something right about it. What your thermoregulation center is doing is ordering a cutdown on the circulation to the extremities of the body. Less blood flowing to them means less heat loss through them, with the heat that is saved going to keep the rest of your body warmer. In situations of outdoor exposure to extreme low temperatures this mechanism increases the danger of frostbitten feet and hands. But the body wisely knows it can, if necessary, suffer the loss of a few fingers or toes and still survive. The vital internal organs, however, must be kept warm or the whole organism will perish.

Cold weather increases urine output. So does caffeine. Everyone seems aware of the fact that it is of vital importance to take in extra water when exercising in hot weather, but they don't realize that they must be just as careful to keep a proper fluid balance during cold weather. Either kind of thermal stress—hot or cold—makes extra demands on the body. The more intense the temperature extreme, and the more active the individual, the more critical proper retention of water in the body becomes.

In too many old movies the just-in-time rescuers, finally coming upon their half-frozen buddy in a snowdrift, promptly proceed to pour a good slug of whiskey down his throat. But alcohol increases the output of urine and thus further upsets the body's balance. And it does something far worse than that: it gives a momentary feeling of warmth as surface blood vessels dilate and the flow of blood to the extremities is increased. Actually the feet and hands are simply being kept warm at the expense of the vital inner core. It is a good idea to avoid exposure to cold after drinking alcohol. If the body's water becomes too depleted, temperatures will soar, the central nervous system is affected, blood plasma volume decreases, and the heart's beat and oxygen-transporting capability are weakened.

Cold and Your Health

What does living in a cold climate do to your health? Well, if you're healthy and young, nothing particularly bad. However, most doctors feel that cold is definitely harmful for many older people. Although some hedged a bit, most tended to agree with the conclusions drawn by the pioneers in their field, Drs. Mills and Petersen, the M.D.'s who pulled no punches in condemning cold climates for the elderly. Cold subjects the human body to stress, particularly if the body is not as resilient as it once was, or if it is beset by illness or physical disabilities.

One of the body's responses to cold is to step up metabolism. That's all right for most people, but for older persons the stress of firing up the system to produce sudden bursts of heat can be too much. If called upon to do this repeatedly, the strain can build up to such an extent that an individual may feel its effects long after a particular episode of exposure to cold has passed.

Doctors and biometeorologists have amassed impressive arrays of statistics to show that the incidence of heart attacks goes up sharply during and after cold spells. Studies that correlated weather with cardiovascular mortality in Memphis and Chicago showed that extremes of temperatures (both hot and cold) were the weather factor most clearly associated with such deaths. Snow was also found to be related to higher heart attack and stroke mortality for a five- to six-day period following the snowfall. Such attacks, when read about in the newspapers, are often assumed to be the result of shoveling snow, but cold-weather heart attacks strike many people who haven't touched a snow shovel.

When a cold wave hits, heart patients aren't the only sick people who can be severely affected. Epileptics experience more seizures, asthmatics suffer more attacks, and arthritis victims must cope with flare-ups of their aches and pains.

"I'm crippled when a cold wave hits," is a common complaint of arthritis patients. Some forms of the broad range of diseases we call arthritis are more aggravated by cold than others. One is the condition called SLE (systemic lupus erythematosus), a kind of arthritis that affects some half a million Americans, mostly women, in a ratio of five females to one male. It involves joint pain, skin rashes, and other symptoms, and the slightest chill can set off an attack.

When it comes to minor ailments—such as migraine headaches and the common cold—biometeorologists also point an accusing finger at cold. Headaches of one kind or another are commonly reported as being triggered or made worse by cold exposure.

"If I step outdoors when the temperature is below freezing I get this terrible headache right away," laments a Minnesota friend. Another acquaintance, living in Vermont, had to give up skiing because of the migraine attacks that invariably hit him on the slopes.

The belief that you're more likely to develop colds and other virus infections during cold spells is not just a bit of folklore. The old saws about not getting your feet wet and not "taking a chill" are founded on fact. Studies at the University of Wisconsin show that when you're subjected to cold, your body temperature can drop slightly. That small drop, though brief, can be enough to encourage the growth of certain previously inactive viruses. They remain dormant, waiting for just the right moment to spring into action. And there you are, coming down with what is called, appropriately, a "cold."

However, almost everybody knows somebody who brags that he or she "never catches cold," in spite of careless flaunting of all the rules about not getting chilled, not getting your feet wet, not stepping out into the cold right after bathing, and so forth.

Some scientific experiments now seem to contradict findings that attribute colds to cold. Dr. Landsberg cites experiments in which groups of people, some kept at ordinary room temperature and others subjected to uncomfortable chilling, were exposed to the common cold virus. There was no appreciable increase in the number of colds in the group of chilled volunteers.

Dr. Harold Brody, a specialist in geriatric medicine at the State University of New York at Buffalo, feels that the suggested daytime 68° F. thermostat setting is not adequate for senior citizens. Prolonged periods of exposure to too-cool temperatures, Dr. Brody points out, can bring about disastrous body changes. Respiration and heartbeat slow down, blood pressure drops, and damage to vital organs, such as the brain, can result. In Britain, where more research has been conducted in this field, it is believed that thousands of elderly people die each year simply because they get too cold!

In the United States, says Dr. Brody, "we do not know the number of people who die of this condition. A medical examiner might not even suspect hypothermia in an elderly patient who has died in bed and might list heart failure as the official cause of death."

Older people and the ill—particularly those suffering from arthritis and asthma—cannot tolerate drastic nighttime drops in temperature. Even though covered with many layers of blankets, they apparently lose body heat through the less well-insulating mattress below them. If the primary consideration were the lives of these individuals, rather than energy consumption, the nighttime thermostat settings in their bedrooms would be 65 for those in the sixty-five to seventy-five age group and 70 for those over the age of seventy-five.

An even greater problem, says Dr. Brody, is that a cold environment can have a devastating psychological effect upon older people, causing them to feel so discouraged and despondent that they stop functioning in any normal fashion and simply take to their beds in an effort to keep warm. Short of such drastic withdrawal, many people who find coping with cold to be too much of a struggle change their life-style, go out less and less, and sink into a slow decline.

Often such people become careless about their diets, subsisting on snack foods that fail to give them the nutrients the body particularly needs in cold weather. Anyone, ill or healthy, invites trouble by ignoring the fact that his body demands more fat in cold weather. Lecithin—which assists in thermoregulation—is another important nutritional need when the weather is cold. To keep warm properly, many people would be better off eating more frequently during the winter months—five small meals a day instead of the usual three. Just the act of breathing causes the body to lose a lot of heat. At a temperature of 68° F., eight calories per hour are lost through breathing. At 24° F., the heat loss is doubled.

Cold and the Medications You Take

Has your doctor ever told you that when the temperature falls below a certain level, you should vary the dosages of medications you are taking? We were shocked by the fact that many of the physicians we talked to had never given any thought to (much less advice to their patients about) the subject of how temperature changes the effect of a given medication.

The following drugs pack more of a wallop in cold weather: analgesics, barbiturates, hallucinogens, monoamine oxidase inhibitors, neuroleptics, narcotics, sulfa drugs, sympatholytics, tetracyclines, tetrahydrocannabinols, and tranquilizers. Dosages of these drugs should probably be decreased during cold spells.

If you aren't sure if any of your regular—or, for that matter, occasionally used—medications fall into the above categories, ask your doctor or your pharmacist. If you find that they do, talk it over with your physician and, if he seems uncertain or disinterested, start wondering if you're going to the right doctor.

Coping with Cold

There are some people who argue that cold is good for them. They may be right—for them. Cold does step up your metabolism and make you feel energetic. It does, under some circumstances, allow you to eat more without gaining weight. It may even be that getting cold does have some beneficial effects—psychological ones at least—if your ethnic heritage is North

European. We know many people of Scandinavian descent who have tried living in California or Florida and who have felt compelled to retreat back to the North.

If you're one of those people who likes cold and lives where it gets cold, and you intend to stay there, you still should not foolishly or dangerously expose yourself to cold. Thousands of Americans a year still succumb to overexposure to cold—the elderly, hunters, hikers, mountain climbers, skiers, motorists stranded in storms, ordinary citizens who didn't feel it was necessary to take a few simple precautions. It doesn't take long to freeze to death. Hands and feet can withstand a drop of thirty to forty degrees below normal body temperature before irreparable damage is done, but if the core temperature of your body drops as little as ten degrees, death can be the result.

If you should suffer exposure to extreme cold, it is essential that you get warmed up as quickly as possible and that you remove any wet clothing immediately. If you are still out in the cold, wet garments will chill you further because of the evaporation from them—not to mention that they might form an icy sheath around your body. Warm liquids (not alcohol) and quick-energy foods like raisins or chocolate will help. Anyone suffering from frostbite should, as soon as possible, be given a warm, not hot, bath. Under no circumstances should frostbitten or frozen parts of the body be rubbed—not with snow, not with warm hands, not with anything. This would further injure already damaged tissues.

How do you know when the cold is too cold for you? By the fact that you're shivering. If you are shivering you are colder than you should permit yourself to be any longer than you have to. One of the problems for the elderly is that their shivering responses are not what they once were. Some elderly persons don't shiver at all and therefore don't even realize they are dangerously chilled.

Before going out and exercising in the cold, you should try to do a few warm-up exercises indoors. The purpose of this is to dilate the arteries to the heart. You should cover your chest area with an extra layer of clothing—like a wool scarf under your jacket—to keep the arteries warm and dilated. Cold can constrict the arteries and quickly cause trouble, especially for those who already have a heart problem.

Scientists calculate that some of the body heat you give up to cold surrounding air comes from your unclothed hands and head, and by the act of breathing. However, 76 percent of the body heat you lose escapes through your clothing. Biometeorologists have invented a handy unit—appropriately called the "Clo" —to measure how effective clothing is at keeping heat in and cold out. One Clo represents the amount of insulation you need when sitting motionless in a room at a temperature of 21° C. (69.8° F.), with an air movement of less than three meters a minute, with a relative humidity of 50 percent. They rate the average man's business suit at one Clo.

The manner in which men and women customarily dress is the source of a fallacious belief that women like—or need—higher room temperatures than men. Some medical people still subscribe to this notion, even though researchers thought they had settled the matter once and for all in the 1940s. They simply dressed men in women's clothing and found that, thus skimpily clad, they too wanted the thermostat set higher. It stands to reason that anyone wearing half a Clo in the way of covering is going to want a warmer temperature than someone wearing a one-Clo suit.

One problem with dressing for cold weather is that it's possible to bundle up too much. Army doctors witnessed a striking example of this when a soldier on Arctic maneuvers collapsed in −40° F. cold and was rushed to the field hospital. The startling diagnosis: heat stroke.

Heat stroke—at 40 below? It happened because of the clothes the soldier was wearing. Frightened by the unfamiliar prospect of doing hard work at such a temperature, the GI had piled on extra layers of underwear and sweaters. He just couldn't bring himself to believe that the doctors knew what they were talking about in recommending that troops wear garments more like the traditional Eskimo parka and trousers.

The Eskimo parka, made of animal skins, hair side in, is so effective at trapping and conserving body heat that it is designed with built-in ventilating areas, with gaps and drawstrings, so that the wearer can periodically get rid of sweat and the excessive heat that builds up. The parka is purposely made short, not much below waist length, so that when its wearer bends over the bare skin of the back is exposed and air can easily flow up under the parka and out the other openings.

Cold and Your Weight

If you suffer from that all-too-common American affliction of being overweight you can take comfort from the fact that outdoor exercise in the cold can help you take off weight faster than would the same activity in warmer temperatures. A group of medical researchers at the University of Toronto exercised six obese men between the ages of twenty-five and forty-six in a cold chamber, with the temperature at $-34°$ C., for three and a half hours on ten successive days. They found the weight loss to be greater than it would have been at normal temperatures, given the same caloric intake and energy output. Furthermore, five of the six kept the weight off after the experiment was discontinued. (The one who regained the weight he had lost was discovered to have been consuming six to seven liters of beer every evening!)

You can feel less guilty about being overweight if you live in a cold climate. The next time someone nags at you to take off some pounds you can cite this fact: doctors have pointed out that the fat layers that obese people have under their skin provide them with extra insulation and protect their bodies from some of the dangers of cold. (Of course, this is hardly an argument for being overweight; the dangers of obesity far outweigh this one minor advantage.)

Escaping the Cold

There are a lot of people who really should get away from the cold as fast as they can. No physician or biometeorologist can say how many, but we believe there are millions of people who needlessly suffer from the cold.

Quite aside from psychological reactions, there are many people who, for sound medical reasons, should definitely consider running away from the cold. We've found almost unanimous medical agreement that these include persons who:

- are allergic to cold (yes, some people actually do have an allergy to cold),
- have certain heart conditions,   2085712
- feel themselves getting "creaky" from the inevitable osteo-arthritis that besets us all if we live long enough,
- have rheumatoid arthritis,
- suffer from certain orthopedic conditions,
- feel themselves harassed by all the problems that go with cold—the snow, the ice, the car troubles, the big utility bills.

If you like cold, or the way of life cold climates provide, and if you don't have any medical condition that's exacerbated by cold weather, fine. But otherwise, if you don't have to, it seems to us the question should be: Why put up with it?

Whatever your reactions to cold, and whether you plan to move away or not, you might be one of the increasing number of northerners who fly off to sunnier climes for winter vacations. A lot of doctors are strongly in favor of such vacations—and a lot of biometeorologists back them up. They're following in the footsteps of Dr. Mills, who long advocated getting away from the stress imposed by cold winters.

However, many physicians have a word of caution. One midwestern physician with whom we've corresponded says, "I doubt that a winter vacation—going from someplace cold to someplace warm—is advisable for everyone. There's considerable shock involved in coming back, and if a person is at all run-down he may well suffer disastrous consequences. We have a saying about going 'from the airport to the hospital,' and it's no joke."

The doctor is right: it's no joke. We've heard essentially the same comment from many other physicians and have seen the statistics that bear out their concern. Records of hospital admissions and mortality rates clearly reflect the hazards of "cold shock." A person comes back tanned and refreshed and instantly finds himself prey to illness from infectious sources or to old chronic afflictions that flare up. Few doctors go so far as to say that it's essential to have a physical check-up before you head south for a winter vacation, but almost all agree that when you get back you should be doubly careful about unnecessary exposure and ease yourself into your cold-weather activities as though your life depended upon it, as indeed it might.

4

Can You Beat the Heat?

Few people like extremely hot weather. Doctors don't like it either, for they are well aware of its effects on the human body. While more people may complain about cold, and feel they suffer more illnesses and aggravations of their ailments in cold weather, the effects of cold are not as devastating as those of heat. In this regard, an even more pertinent question than "Should you run away from the cold?" is "Can you beat the heat?"

The Menace of Heat

From January 14 to 19, 1965, New York City was blanketed under six inches of snow, in the grip of a severe cold wave during which temperatures dropped to 4° F. and winds averaged 25 mph. Deaths soared, with one of the boroughs reporting a mortality rate 67 percent above normal for the period.

Alarming as those statistics seem, they don't begin to compare with what happened in New York City when it sweltered in 105° F. temperatures during the summer of the following year. On the Fourth of July, 1966, deaths in New York more than doubled. In one borough, Queens, they almost tripled. Heat syndrome itself was not listed as a cause of death by New York's

Department of Health. The "causes" with the most startling increases were: cancer, up 128 percent; atherosclerotic heart disease, up 161 percent; stroke, up 176 percent; and influenza and pneumonia, which most of us tend to think of as wintertime illnesses, *up 315 percent!*

The country's midsection was also experiencing record heat that summer. In St. Louis, where a maximum temperature of 106° F. was reached, the mortality rate went up *524 percent!* Heat syndrome *was* recognized as a cause of death there; it was held accountable for 28 percent of the deaths that occurred. The other causes: cancer, up 100 percent above the expected rate; atherosclerotic heart disease, up 162 percent; influenza and pneumonia, up 350 percent.

Heat, in other words, can be a killer. It is a killer to which not many of us give much thought. William Hodges, of the National Climatic Center, in referring to the more than 1,500 people who died because of the excessive heat experienced in the northeastern states in August 1975, says, "Strangely, this catastrophe has been taken largely as a matter of course."

Short of actually threatening your life, heat can make you mighty sick, assailing you with what is medically known as "heat-caused disorders." Many of these disorders are merely annoying, but some are serious. According to Dr. Felix Sulman, an Israeli biometeorologist, they include:

Prickly heat, a stinging rash that hits its victims mostly on humid, hot days when skin glistens with sweat. It's caused by skin bacteria attacking minute skin sores.

Heat edema, the swelling of the extremities, particularly the feet and ankles, most likely to occur after several days of great heat. This condition is a product of histamine and the hormone serotonin produced in the body.

Water depletion heat stress, occurring when you don't replace the water you're losing in sweat. It is accompanied by symptoms of fatigue, dizziness, fever, and finally delirium.

Salt depletion heat exhaustion, which can create a host of disagreeable symptoms as salt is carried away in sweat. Fatigue, nausea, and cramps can occur when sodium in your blood is replaced by potassium from body cells.

Heat cramps, muscle spasms that can occur when you're doing hard work in extreme heat and are drinking large amounts of water but not replacing salt. The mineral concentration of the blood changes, and a sort of tug-of-war occurs between minerals that have differing effects on muscles. Potassium and magnesium decrease muscle contractions; sodium and calcium increase them.

Heat syncope (heat exhaustion), a condition in which so much blood is drawn to the skin that the brain fails to receive its necessary blood supply. The result is collapse, one of the dangerous possible consequences of strenuous exercise in extreme heat.

Heat stroke, the most serious of all the heat-caused disorders, which can be fatal. It can befall the unwary in any climate, in Maine or Montana as much as in Alabama or Arizona. It's literally a "stroke" brought on by exercise on a hot day—not necessarily an extremely hot one—or by simple exposure to very great heat. It's a result of a rise in body temperature to 107° F. or 42° C.—the point where the thermoregulation system breaks down, with possible brain injury and death. Dr. W. Jack Stelmach, president of the American Academy of Family Physicians (in 1979), estimates that heat stroke may be fatal in 50 percent of the cases.

"Heat stroke is much more common than is realized," report meteorologists J. T. McLaughlin and M. D. Shulman, of Rutgers, the State University, in New Jersey. Medical authorities agree. Even when a doctor is called or the patient is rushed to the hospital, the examining physician may not correctly identify the illness. Doctors frequently diagnose heat stroke as heart failure, cerebral hemorrhage, spinal meningitis, or even Rocky Mountain spotted fever.

How Your Body Keeps Its Cool

You are a homeothermal creature: your body, if it is healthy, maintains its temperature at a constant level in spite of the air temperatures, hot or cold, to which it is subjected. If you come in from a cold winter day or a hot summer one and take your temperature, it will always be close to 98.6° F. (37° C.) if you are in good health. The body manages this feat by keeping its heat gain and its heat loss in balance. The body is constantly both gaining and losing heat. It gains heat in three ways: by producing it in the body (through various metabolic processes), by taking it up from the environment, and by exercising. The body also loses heat in three ways: by radiation (giving up heat to cooler objects or surroundings), by conduction and convection to the air when its temperature is lower than that of the body (air molecules in contact with the skin are warmed, move away, and cooler ones come in to take their place, are in turn warmed, and so on), and by evaporation (in other words, sweating). When the air surrounding you is warmer than your skin, sweating is your only means of cooling off.

The 2.5 million corkscrew-like channels in your skin can push out an astonishing quantity of liquid. Tests by the army in the Arizona desert showed that sweltering GIs lost an average of a quart an hour. On an ordinary hot summer day in the Northeast, with exertion no greater than that demanded by the act of walking across a golf course, you can lose as much as a pint an hour. You're probably not conscious of all the sweating you're doing; insensible sweating goes on all the time.

In the Southwest we've heard many people remark that one reason they like the dry climate is that they "don't sweat." Of course they sweat; if they didn't they would die. However, the dry air absorbs the sweat before it has time to form visible beads of moisture or soak through clothing.

How much cooling you need and how much water your body loses through sweating depends, of course, on what you are doing. Persons engaging in hard physical work sweat three times as much as persons doing desk work in an environment of the same temperature.

In addition to those amazing sweat glands, the human body

comes equipped with a truly fantastic set of other devices that regulate its temperature. Though you may be unconscious of the watchful efforts of the thermoregulatory system, it is as necessary to your survival as is your heart, your lungs, or any other vital organ. Fortunately, for most of us most of the time this remarkable life-sustaining mechanism continues to work, withstanding assaults from within and without.

Your responses to the temperature of the air around you start in a network of sensors in your skin. These sensitive nerve ends have been called "biothermometers." There are two kinds of them, one responding to heat, the other to cold. Both kinds are more plentiful in certain parts of the body. Nipples, chest, nose, upper arm and forearm, and the surface of the abdomen are the most sensitive parts. The face, hands, scalp, and mucous membranes are the least sensitive, because they have the fewest receptors. So delicate are these sensors that they are capable of detecting temperature differences as small as one-fifth of one centigrade degree in the air meeting the skin.

The sensors continually relay their temperature reports to thermoregulation centers in the brain, one of them in the hypothalamus, the other in the cerebral cortex. Acting on this information, the centers send out signals to produce the hormones that affect metabolism, the rate at which your body converts food to energy. The center in the hypothalamus contains two distinct mechanisms: one prevents overheating, the other protects against too much cooling.

There are people who aren't bothered much by heat. In fact, there are some who seem to thrive on it, although not on truly excessive heat, the kind that gives rise to hyperthermia (heat stroke). Individual responses differ widely. Your hormonal system, your state of health, your degree of weather sensitivity, and the frequency of your exposure to heat are all factors that may keep you from "feeling the heat" at levels that disturb other people.

Your body build probably has a lot to do with how you react

to heat. We say "probably" because biometeorologists are still exploring the subject, with differing results. In tests carried out in the climate chamber of Penn State's Laboratory for Human Performance Research, where subjects walked on a treadmill at various air temperatures and various speeds, it was concluded that "body size appeared to exert little influence on the amount of thermal strain." However, when the subjects engaged in more strenuous activities, different body builds appeared to have considerable influence. Obese women are under much greater heat strain than thinner women, but, surprisingly, small men seem to be less tolerant of heat than men of normal size and weight. Children are much more affected by extreme heat than are adults.

Getting Adjusted to Heat

It isn't just the torrid heat of summer that causes problems. Many persons, particularly heart patients, find early summer, the first warm days of the season, the time of greatest discomfort and hazard. This is also the time when people are most likely to succumb to the onslaughts of "weekend syndrome." Those who haven't had any strenuous exercise in months feel the urge to get out onto the golf course or the tennis court. Not only are they out of shape, but they haven't had time to become adjusted to the heat. Though some of the collapses of sedentary workers who suddenly subject themselves to unaccustomed physical strain are caused by heart attacks, many result from heat exhaustion.

Dr. Ralph F. Goldman, of the U.S. Army Research Institute of Environmental Medicine at Natick, Massachusetts, explains how heat exhaustion can result when an individual continues to work or play in heat beyond the level of acute discomfort: "The heart rate accelerates in an attempt to maintain blood pressure and supply blood to the brain. However, at a heart rate of about 180 beats per minute, there is inadequate time between beats for filling the chambers of the heart for the next beat. Thereafter, heart rate increases explosively as, with each beat, cardiac output falls as a bit less blood is pumped. The individual will faint or 'black out.' "

Dr. Goldman suggests that, to become acclimatized to exercising in the heat, you should start by doing no more than 100 minutes of exercise a day. After the first day, a healthy person should experience a 30-percent improvement in his performance and ability to stand the heat. The improvement increases dramatically and should be about 95 percent after a week. Such a program will condition the cardiovascular system as well as the sweat secretion and sodium conservation mechanisms. It is important to keep it up for, as Dr. Goldman points out, "heat acclimatization, once induced, can be maintained by as little as once a week exposure to working in the heat but otherwise diminishes slowly over a two- to three-week period and disappears thereafter." In other words, if you stop for a few weeks, you have to start your conditioning program all over again!

The sudden onset of hot weather also necessitates changes in the kind of clothes you are wearing, and adjustments in diet and water intake that you make slowly and almost without planning in years when you slide more gradually into summer heat. You may still be eating foods better fitted for colder weather and not drinking enough liquids to take care of the stepped-up water loss that comes with higher temperatures.

Everyone is affected in some degree by the adjustments the body must make from cold to heat and from heat to cold, even when the transition is a gradual one. What cold-climate dweller hasn't experienced spring fever, with its draggy feeling of total fatigue? While it isn't a "fever," it has very real symptoms for very real physical reasons.

When the weather gets warm, your body tries to adjust to the new outside temperature by dilating the blood vessels so that more blood can be carried to the skin surface, where evaporative cooling will reduce body temperature. This process calls for more blood, which your body goes to work to produce. First it makes more plasma; other components will be added later. So, literally, your blood is "thinner" for a time. Many bodily forces have to be marshaled to produce the extra blood, and until it is sufficient to meet the new demands, you'll experience the lassitude we call spring fever.

We would all be better off if spring came gradually and each day became warmer by a fraction of a degree until summer's heat peak was reached, and if after that each day were just a little cooler than the one preceding it until, once again, we were back to the year's lowest temperatures. Weather, however, doesn't work in such an orderly fashion. Extremes of temperature are often thrown at us unexpectedly, before we've had time to prepare ourselves for them.

What happened during an East Coast heat wave in late September 1970 illustrates the life-and-death importance of acclimatization to heat. In Washington, D.C., the death rate climbed, but not as much as it did in New York City. The reason was simple. Washingtonians had been suffering through uncomfortably hot weather all along, while New Yorkers had been enjoying pleasantly cool weather before the onset of the heat wave.

Heat and Performance

Nobody, no matter how long he lives where it is excessively hot most of the time, ever really functions at his best when temperatures are high. Ellsworth Huntington, the pioneering MIT bioclimatologist, pointed out that even the Javanese, an equatorial people who live where temperatures are commonly 80° F. or higher, enjoy better health and greater energy when they move to higher altitudes where the temperature averages 70° F. or lower.

"In a general way," said Huntington, "we may say that a mean temperature of about 63° F. for day and night together is the optimum for physical well-being in man and that the optimum rarely rises above 70° F. even among people who live in the hottest parts of the world."

Excessive heat makes you physically sluggish; it also impairs your mental efficiency, slows your reaction time, and hampers your ability to deal with stress.

The validity of such comments as "It seems like I'm all thumbs when it's hot" has been amply proved by many laboratory observations. One classic experiment was carried out by Dr. Mills at the University of Cincinnati. In his laboratory there he tested three groups of rats for their ability to make their way through a maze under different temperature conditions. Those in the first group, at 65° F., required twelve trials to get the prize of food awaiting them at the end of the maze. The second group, operating at 76° F., needed twenty-six trials. The rats in the third group, subjected to an uncomfortable 90° F., required forty-eight runs, and many failed to make it at all.

Dr. Mills later made observations that confirmed his conclusion that higher temperatures have a definite effect on mental capacities—not only of rats but of humans. Various IQ and mathematics tests given under controlled room temperatures showed marked slowdowns in the speed at which participants solved problems. Also, scores were lower.

Heat, Medicines, and Alcohol

Heat changes the way we respond to various medications, just as cold does. Physicians report difficulty in establishing proper dosages of drugs given for hypertension in the summer months because blood pressure tends to drop in warm weather. A drug designed to reduce the high blood pressure of the hypertensive patient may have just the desired effect in the cold winter months, whereas the same dosage taken during the heat of summer might have too great an effect.

Medical researchers admit they have a long way to go before they have established a truly accurate profile of how hundreds of common drugs behave in different seasons, but dosages of the following drugs should probably be decreased in hot weather: anticoagulants, antihypertensives, anti-Parkinson's disease drugs, antispasmodics, atropine-like drugs, cortisone-like drugs, mono-amine oxidase inhibitors, neuroleptics, parasympathomimetics, phenothiazines, sedatives, sleep inducers, thiazide diuretics, tranquilizers.

There are even a few drugs, such as antibiotics, antidepressants, and antidiuretics, that you should decrease the use of if you are going to be out in the sunshine. If you must take them, you should avoid being out in the sun.

If you take any of these drugs, consult your doctor about varying dosages of them as the weather gets hot, or if you're leaving a cold climate for a winter vacation in a warm one.

One fact nobody can dispute is that alcohol is more intoxicating in summer than it is when the weather is cold. On an extremely hot day in midsummer one bottle of beer may have the alcoholic punch of two in the winter. The explanation is that warm nervous tissues absorb alcohol quickly, getting it into the bloodstream before your body has time to burn it.

How to Handle the Heat

If you live in a climate where temperatures soar, it's pretty hard to avoid some exposure to excessive heat. Even if you enjoy air-conditioned comfort much of the time, there are occasions when you must venture out of your cool sanctuary—home, office, factory, or car—if only to walk across parking lots. And, in a society increasingly conscious of, and striving for, physical fitness, millions who might previously have shunned the outdoors when it was uncomfortably hot are now out there jogging, golfing, and playing tennis.

Whatever your life-style, you're bound to find yourself exposed to the vagaries of the weather. The very fact that your exposure is brief and sporadic may make the effects of heat even more detrimental than they were to people of previous generations who put up with heat more of the time.

Doctors we have talked to about air conditioning have pointed out some of the problems it creates. A Los Angeles physician told us, "It's a good thing we're being asked to maintain our indoor summertime temperatures at 78 to 80, instead of the 72, or even 70, that many people have kept their homes and offices at in recent years. The shock of going out into 100-degree heat—or even 90-degree heat—from such low temperatures is hard on you. It's better to be a little hotter all the time than to take that kind of punishment. And the reverse is just as bad—coming in all hot and sweaty from outside into 70-degree temperatures can give you a sudden chill and make you susceptible to illness."

Dr. Kenneth L. Benfer, of the Department of Internal Medicine, York Hospital, York, Pennsylvania, is just one of the many psysicians who worry about the effects of "thermal shock" on their patients. Among the cases he cites are those of a surgeon who developed acute frontal sinusitis from going out into extreme outdoor heat after spending his days in an air-conditioned hospital; an elderly arthritic who, after sitting through a program in an air-conditioned auditorium, was unable to walk when he stepped out into 95-degree heat; and an insurance salesman who worked in an air-conditioned office and who, when he went out into the heat, suffered severe chest pains and had to be rushed to the hospital.

We met one woman who takes a truly drastic approach to avoiding "thermal shock." "I just don't go outside all summer," she announced.

She lives in an apartment high up in "Big John," the John Hancock building in Chicago. In the morning she descends in an elevator to a lower-floor office where she works as a junior executive. For lunch she goes to a restaurant on another floor. She shops in stores on various levels. For an evening's entertainment she can go to one of the theaters in the same building. It's the kind of totally controlled indoor existence science-fiction writers have long written about.

What does living like that do to the human physiology? What would happen to our Chicago friend if she *had* to venture outside the great cocoon of Big John? Outside, where, in spite of the alleviating breezes off Lake Michigan, the temperature can get to

100° F. or above and the humidity can be a dripping 85 percent or so?

"Well, so far I haven't had to find out," this particular heat hater told us.

"The effect could be devastating," commented a doctor we talked to. "It would be a terrible shock to her system. I hope she has a strong heart."

"You know, there's a great deal to be said for trying to live with the weather," he went on to say. "People used to do it."

How *did* they do it, back in the good old days? First of all, they built their houses and other buildings to take full advantage of any cooling breezes. They drew the drapes or blinds on the sunny windows and opened up the others. And they used fans to move the air. As long as air is moving, you can stand it being pretty hot.

In air-conditioned buildings today the air is almost motionless. If the extra energy consumed in a heat wave brings about a "brownout" and the air-conditioning systems fail, temperatures inside buildings that are wholly dependent on air conditioning to make them habitable can become intolerable. During the September 1970 heat wave in Washington, D.C., people who lived in old-fashioned apartments and houses that were not air-conditioned but that took advantage of air movement—artificial or natural—were able to cope. Many of the residents of, or workers in, air-conditioned buildings were forced to leave their homes and offices and take to the streets and parks.

Of course, for all the problems air conditioning presents, it is certainly here to stay. And who would want it otherwise? For many of us—for infants, whose thermoregulatory control is not yet stable; for the ill, particularly those with heart disease; and for the elderly—air conditioning is, quite literally, a lifesaver. In general, older people fare better in climates that are warm year-round than they do in colder climates, even though they have to stay indoors in air-conditioned environments for those periods that are too hot. After all, even those parts of the United States that we consider "cold" are subject to searing summer heat waves. There is almost no place that doesn't have excessive heat at times. Even Alaska can get unbearably hot.

Altitude, of course, can make a crucial difference. In the Southwest, which is largely desert, the inhabitants of the high-altitude mountain areas can almost wholly escape uncomfortable heat. And, as such lucky people like to point out, no matter how hot their days are, their nights are always cool.

"I can take any amount of heat in the daytime as long as it cools off at night," is a commonly heard statement. Those who feel that way may be more right than even they realize. Dr. Herbert M. Austin, of the National Oceanic and Atmospheric Administration (NOAA), points out that maximum nighttime temperatures may be even more important than are the daytime highs. Night is a time for the body to recuperate, and high temperatures during the hours of rest can prevent it from doing so. Cool temperatures at night, on the other hand, can give the body the chance it needs to reestablish its heat balance.

Certainly, no matter where you live, you can protect yourself from some of the worst effects of torrid temperatures if you follow a few simple rules:

Slow down. Your body is already under stress; don't subject it to extra strain.

Heed your body's early warning signals. At the first sign of weakness, dizziness, nausea, or any other unusual symptom, immediately reduce your level of activity and get to someplace where it's cool.

Eat properly. Smaller meals and lighter foods will help you weather the heat. While you still need protein foods, go easier on them, for they increase metabolic heat production and water loss.

Drink plenty of water. You are losing a lot of water and it must be replaced.

Don't get too much sun. Sunburn makes the job of heat dissipation that much more difficult.

Avoid thermal shock. Acclimate yourself gradually to warmer weather. Treat yourself extra gently for those first critical hot days. Don't set your air conditioner to deliver too low a temperature.

Vary your thermal environment. Physical stress increases with exposure time in heat-wave weather. Try to get out of the heat for at least a few hours each day.

Dress properly. Wear lightweight, loose-fitting, light-colored clothing. Clothing creates a vapor barrier around the body, impeding the evaporation of sweat. Women in general do better than men at dressing for summer. Fashion still dictates that men wear complete business suits in their offices, and on the street going to and from their offices, even though the temperature may be over 100. Actually, in hot weather you should wear as little clothing as is possible—or permissible.

5

Humidity and the Dry-Climate Mystique

Almost everybody hates humidity. Yet, in several tests aimed at finding out how well people can detect humidity, it was found that most people are very poor judges of humidity when temperatures are moderate. When temperatures are cold they're only slightly more accurate with their estimates. It is only when both the temperature and the relative humidity are very high that people do noticeably better at judging humidity, and even then they simply know that it is "high." The reason they know that comes down simply to the fact that they are uncomfortable. It is an amazing physiological fact that the human body has no humidity sensors, only receptors that react to cold and heat.

If the air surrounding it is dry enough, the human body can withstand an astounding level of heat. In climate-chamber tests, with the relative humidity at almost zero, men have been able to take—for very short periods of time, of course—oven-like heats of 250° F.!

As we said in the preceding chapter, when the air around you is hotter than you are, your body's way of cooling off is to produce sweat. Sweating, however, only helps you if the moisture your skin gives off can evaporate. If there is already so much water in the ambient air that your sweat can't evaporate and instead just trickles down your brow, sweating doesn't help. You are losing water for no good purpose—an uncomfortable, and sometimes dangerous, situation. It's easy to see why you don't mind the heat as much in a dry climate, or on an unusually dry day, even though the temperature may be very high. The sweat you give off evaporates as fast as you can produce it. You have become, in effect, an evaporative cooler.

What Is Relative Humidity?

The words *relative humidity* are used to describe the amount of water *actually* in a given volume of air as it compares with the amount of moisture that volume of air *could* hold.

For example, one cubic foot of air, at a temperature of 70° F., *can* hold eight grains of water. (A grain of water is 1/7000 of a pound.) If that cubic foot of air *actually* contains two grains (or one-fourth of what it *could* hold), the relative humidity is 25 percent.

The amount of water the air can hold varies with atmospheric pressure and temperature. Warm air can hold a lot more water than cold air can. When the barometer reads 30 and the thermometer 0° F., a cubic foot of air can hold about half a grain of vapor per cubic foot. At 32° F., it can hold two grains; at 100° F., about twenty grains. So, when it's 90° F. in the shade and the relative humidity is reported as 80 percent, the air is holding a lot of water, quantitatively as well as relatively.

The relative humidity to which you are subjected changes from day to day and from hour to hour, and it varies even more from place to place. Readings taken in adjacent regions can show great disparities at any given time. U.S. Weather Service studies often register differences as great as 15 percent within a few miles, or even a few blocks. And when you compare the relative humidity of the space outside your front door with that immediately inside the same door, you will find, particularly during those months when your home is heated, that there can be dramatic variations in humidity in the space of just a few inches.

The T-HI—Measure of Comfort

To measure the effects of the temperature-humidity combination, meteorologists devised the T-HI, the Temperature-Humidity Index. It's arrived at by combining the temperatures of a dry-bulb thermometer (the kind we're all familiar with) with those of a wet-bulb thermometer. A wet-bulb thermometer is one in which the mercury-containing bulb is covered with a woven cloth that serves as a wick to draw water from a reservoir. This water evaporates at a rate corresponding to the dryness of the air.

The formula for arriving at the T-HI is T-HI $= 0.4(td + tw)$ $+ 15$, with td standing for the dry-bulb temperature and tw for the wet-bulb temperature (in degrees Fahrenheit). Suppose that the dry-bulb reading is 90° F. and the wet-bulb reading 80° F. The T-HI would then be 83. This is neither a temperature reading nor a relative humidity reading, but it does indicate very accurately the comfort level of the humidity-temperature combination.

What is an ideal T-HI? It has been found, from thousands of observations in and out of climate chambers, that at a T-HI of 71 nearly everybody is comfortable. As soon as the reading begins to drop below this level some people start to feel too cool. When it hits 67 almost everyone feels chilly. When the T-HI starts to climb above 71 some people at once feel discomfort; at 80 almost everybody feels miserable. Levels above 85 can cause dangerous physical reactions. Heat stroke, for example, occurs most often at T-HI readings above 85.

High T-HI's affect you mentally as well as physically, reducing your mental alertness and efficiency. In tests of college students, it was found that typists were 10 to 20 percent slower in a hot room with high humidity than they were in an equally hot room with low humidity. A test with a group of telegraph operators in England clearly showed the results of high T-HI's. In climate chambers where the relative humidity was high the temperature was gradually raised as the operators took down Morse code dictation over the telephone. At 85° F. they made an average of 12 mistakes an hour. At 100° F. that went up to 17.3 mistakes. At 105° F. (by which time the T-HI had climbed to 89), the mistakes took a huge jump—to 94.7 an hour.

Humidity Can Make You Sick

Hospital admissions rise, as does the mortality rate, during humid heat spells and during cold waves when the humidity is high. How much of the problem is due to humidity and how much to the excessive heat or cold, or to combinations of weather factors, biometeorologists aren't sure.

The dire effects due to weather are related not so much to the exact measurements or readings of these weather phenomena but to *changes* in all three of them. (Humidity can't be divorced from other weather factors. Under certain circumstances a given relative humidity will create problems, but under others the same humidity level will cause no trouble at all.)

For instance, when medical researchers try to discover a correlation between arthritis flare-ups and periods of extremely high relative humidity, they fail to conclude that a given level of relative humidity at a given temperature and a given atmospheric pressure is conducive to distress in arthritis patients.

Researchers express no confusion, however, about the part humidity plays in spreading microorganisms that cause illness. When someone with the flu or a cold sneezes, tiny virus-laden droplets are sprayed into the air. Under some conditions, these contaminated droplets can float for some time before they fall to the ground or the floor. High humidity helps them survive longer at levels where they may be inhaled by potential new victims.

Dr. Helmut Landsberg explains: "In air with low relative humidity, the droplets will evaporate and leave the microorganisms without a base of fluid, which it needs for survival. High humidities prevent this evaporation and keep the droplet intact."

The behavior of viruses and other organisms in the air is modified by temperature. At very cold temperatures, water droplets, even though they continue to float, present an inhospitable environment for viruses. When the droplets freeze, they cease to be a swimming pool for microbes. This is a factor in the low incidence of colds in the Arctic. It's also the reason why you're very unlikely to catch a cold out on the ski runs in the winter. Cold sufferers may be coughing all around you without doing you any harm because the viruses are inactivated by the freezing droplets.

Should You Move to a Dry Climate?

The very week in which we are writing this particular chapter is one in which New Mexico is experiencing record-breaking temperatures. Yet most of the time we don't even turn on the air conditioner. Why? Because the relative humidity has been down around 5 *percent!* There are other factors in the climate of the Southwest to which health improvements can be attributed, but almost everyone agrees that the one that makes the real difference is the dry air.

For well over a hundred years people have been moving to the southwestern part of the United States in search of health. First it was the victims of tuberculosis, some of whom were bedded down in wagons and carried west. And, once the railroad made the trip easier, every train brought its share of health seekers. Many who tried did not survive the trip; some were so sick they didn't last long once they got to the promised land; but many others, in spite of the fact that they had been given "five years" or "one year" or "six months at the most" by their doctors back home, regained their health and lived to ripe old ages.

One of the early migrants was Josiah Gregg, who arrived in New Mexico in 1831. He wrote glowingly of the health benefits to be found in the Southwest, and among his writings is this much-quoted gem: "The old people look older than they do in any other country. There is a local proverb that the region is so healthful that the inhabitants never die; but lean, attenuated and wrinkled, like Egyptian mummies, dry up ultimately and are blown away."

There are disadvantages, of course, to living in very dry climates. You may have to change your ways of doing things—like tending to your lawn and garden chores in the morning and evening, and staying out of the intense sun during the midday hours. The sun can even be a menace to light-skinned people, increasing their chances of developing skin cancer if they fail to use good judgment as to the amount of exposure they get.

Another problem is that once you have adapted to a dry climate, it is harder to return to humid ones for visits or vacations, especially during times of the year when it's likely to be both humid and hot.

Most people we've talked to are convinced that the advantages far outweigh the disadvantages. Sinuses are not swollen, breathing passages aren't clogged, and respiratory problems often seem to vanish. The spores and molds that cause so many allergic reactions in damp climates cannot survive in the dry air and soil. And the combination of sun, warmth, and dryness often does wonders for other ailments, including arthritis.

Thousands of southwesterners are here for health reasons. And thousands more—judging by the stories one hears—came for reasons other than health but were surprised and gratified to find themselves feeling better, or even getting well. We are constantly reminded of Mark Twain's classic remark: "I know a man who came to Nevada to die. But he made a failure of it."

Of course, to many transplanted easterners, the Southwest seems stark and forbidding, especially at first. Familiar with countryside that is predominantly green, they find it hard to get used to the fact that in the Southwest it is the cities, where trees and lawns are planted and given plenty of water, that are bright, verdant oases in the desert. Outside the inhabited areas, the landscape stretches away in sun-baked brownness. To be sure, there are mountainous regions that are as green in summer, as golden in the fall, and as snowy in the winter as forested areas anywhere, but, by and large, the Southwest is an arid land, with many localities getting less than ten inches of rain a year.

In the United States the dry climates are all found in the West, particularly in the Southwest—in west Texas, New Mexico, Arizona, Colorado, Utah, Nevada, and much of southern California. There are also dry climates, although colder ones, farther north in the West—up through all the Rocky Mountain states. Even the eastern portions of Oregon and Washington are dry.

6

Sunlight and
Your Health

Millions of people soak up the sun on summer beaches, head south for winter vacations, and speak wistfully of moving to a sunny climate. Millions more have actually up and moved to the Sunbelt. They all attest to the fact that we're a nation of sun worshipers. Most of us staunchly believe that sunlight striking our epidermis has magic properties beneficial to both body and mind. If you're among those who subscribe to this philosophy, you'll be happy to know that the biometeorologists go right along with you. Their research has revealed that the benefits of sunlight are all they're supposed to be—and more.

Sunlight can not only make you feel good, but can help make you well. In the new science called phototherapy, medicine has found a tool with great potential for treating several diseases. Many medical authorities agree with the prediction made by Thomas P. Vogl of Columbia Presbyterian Medical Center in New York, who, commenting on the healing power of light, says, "Light will become as important as drugs."

What Sunlight Does to You

Does a sunny day give you a lift? Probably. And it's probable, too, that your moods are determined more by your reaction to sunlight than they are by any other single weather factor—even atmospheric pressure, which has such a notable impact on your psyche.

One effect biometeorologists have discovered is that a sunny day alters your perception of other weather factors. In an experiment carried out in Canada, designed to see if people can judge humidity, it was found that the subjects taking part in the study were sure that the air was "dry" when the sun was shining. At the same humidity and temperature levels, they thought the air was "humid" when the sun wasn't shining. Other experiments have shown that a cold winter day is perceived as "warmer" when the sun is shining, even though the subjects have not been directly exposed to the sun.

Researchers admit that they're somewhat baffled as to just why the sun has a benign psychological effect, although they know perfectly well that it does. Studies have shown that persons who are mentally disturbed are more so when skies are overcast. For example, one study made by the Biometeorological Research Centre in the Netherlands determined that the period of greatest disturbance for mentally ill people occurred in November and December, the two months with the least sunlight.

Mentally healthy people are influenced by the presence or absence of sunlight as much as mentally disturbed people, although the effects are not so noticeable.

There are sound medical reasons why sunlight can alter the way you feel. It causes numerous physiological effects. Researchers have determined that sunlight acts upon:

The circulatory system. Exposure to sunlight causes a drop in blood pressure, with the greatest drop occurring in healthy young adults. This is due to the release of histamine in the skin, causing the capillaries to dilate and thereby receive more blood. When you feel slowed down and sleepy on a beach this is one of the reasons why.

The gastrointestinal tract. Ultraviolet exposure can speed up the secretion of gastric juices. (This is one reason why badly sunburned persons can feel quite ill.)

The blood. Numerous changes take place in the blood when you are exposed to the ultraviolet in sunlight. One of them is a marked increase in the number of red blood cells and of hemoglobin. An increase in white cells has also been observed.

Metabolism. Protein metabolism is increased by exposure to sunlight. In some people this results in increased energy, as indicated by work output studies utilizing the ergometer.

And, of course, *the skin,* where sunlight converts a chemical substance in the skin into the vitamin D your body needs.

It is possible that there are other bodily responses to sunlight that science has not yet discovered. You have a pea-sized gland at the base of your brain, for instance, that has long baffled medical science. It was called the "seat of the soul" by René Descartes, the seventeenth-century philosopher and scientist. Physiologists, up to quite recently, could do no better than term it "the mystery gland." They knew it had something to do with light perception, but since they were unable to establish any function it performed in the body, they dismissed it as a vestigial organ, a "third eye" that may once have had some usefulness but that no longer had a purpose.

It was not until 1958 that researchers discovered that not only does the pineal gland react to light, it also produces a hormone, melatonin, as a result of that response. The amount of this hormone in the body varies at different times of the day. Melatonin is known to induce sleep, inhibit ovulation, and modify the body's secretion of other hormones. The exploration of all the effects of this hormone is still a frontier of medicine, termed "the nascent field of clinical pinealogy" by Dr. Richard Wurtman, of the Harvard Medical School and the Massachusetts Institute of Technology (MIT).

The Dangers of Too Much Sun

There are dangers in sunlight, too, the most common hazard being sunburn. Dr. Wurtman points out that "sunburn is largely an affliction of industrial civilizations. If people could expose themselves to sunlight for one or two hours every day, weather permitting, their skin's reaction to the gradual erythemal [skin-reddening] solar radiation that occurs during late winter and spring would provide them with a protective layer of pigmentation for withstanding ultraviolet radiation of summer intensities."

This is a scientist's way of saying that after you have gone through a winter and spring without much exposure to sun, you are most susceptible to sunburn, since you haven't built up any protective coat of tan.

You don't see many sunburned people in the sunnier portions of the Sunbelt because they've garnered one of the bonuses of living in a sunny climate. Even the most cloistered inhabitant of an air-conditioned office building gets a lot more sun than his compatriots in the cloudier North. On journeys to and from work, during lunch breaks, and on weekends, the sunny-climate dweller automatically picks up a lot of hours of exposure.

For the unconditioned, pallid northerner, it's those first days of reveling out in the springtime sun that are the most danger-ous. It takes only a few minutes to get uncomfortably sunburned and only an hour or two to acquire a really dangerous burn. Anyone can be hit by sunburn—black-, brown-, and red-skinned people as well as those with lighter skin. However, the 850 million white-skinned people on this planet have most of the problems with sunburn, while the almost 2 billion nonwhites don't have to worry as much.

The skin of dark-skinned people contains more melanin, a chemical that limits the energy of the sunlight penetrating it. Melanin, whose production is stimulated by sunlight, screens out the sunburn-causing wavelengths. The process of melanin production begins almost immediately upon exposure to sunlight and builds up with repeated exposure.

Even among light-skinned people there is a great difference in susceptibility to sunburn. Photosensitivity, to use the medical term, varies with age, sex, and complexion. The lightest-complexioned people, particularly those with red hair, sunburn quickly. Young children are least likely to sunburn, followed by adults over fifty. Far more males are photosensitive, although women during the first days of the menstrual cycle and during pregnancy are more photosensitive than they are at other times. And, finally, different parts of the body sunburn at different rates. The breasts are the most photosensitive area of the body, followed in order by the abdomen, back, cheeks, arms, and legs.

The most dangerous reaction to ultraviolet is, of course, the development of skin cancer. The radiation can damage cells in those susceptible to this malignancy, creating lesions in the skin. Most subject to this form of cancer are people of North European ethnic background who spend much time outdoors, especially in sunny climates. Skin cancer is ten times more common in Texas (2,000 cases per million population) than it is in North Dakota (200 per million).

Are You Losing Needed Sunlight?

While sunlight can be harmful if you're not careful about your exposure to it, it is, of course, essential to life and health. A current concern on the part of scientists is that we may not be getting enough of it. For, wherever you live, whether in the Frostbelt or the Sunbelt, in the city, the suburbs, or the country, you're getting less sunlight than people in the same locality did in the past.

The reason? Air pollution is affecting the amount of sunlight reaching the earth. Scientists at the Mount Wilson Observatory in California report a 10-percent loss in sunlight intensity in the last half-century. A Smithsonian Institution study indicates the loss may be even greater elsewhere. It puts the loss at 14 percent in the last sixty years. Loss of the ultraviolet part of the spectrum is even greater. Large urban areas have been found to have 30 percent less than nearby rural countryside.

"If air pollution continues to get worse, perhaps we may soon be wearing aluminum collars to reflect the diminishing sunlight. The loss of ten to fourteen percent of visible sunlight and even more of ultraviolet is frightening." This is the expression of concern by a scientist who has made amazing discoveries about the power of sunlight and the dangers of screening it out. This light authority is Dr. John Ott, the developer of time-lapse photography. (You've seen the results of his work in Walt Disney films in which flowers apparently burst into bloom in a few seconds.)

John Ott's years of experience with special-effects lighting had taught him a lot about the way plants respond to light. An unusual personal experience led him to some exciting thoughts about what light might be doing to humans.

An arthritis sufferer, Ott had to walk with a cane. Because he often worked outdoors in bright light, he wore sunglasses much of the time. One day his sunglasses broke and, before Ott got around to replacing them, he began to notice an improvement in his arthritic condition. Few, if any, people would have seen a connection, but because Ott was used to thinking about the effects of light, it occurred to him that his arthritis might be better because he wasn't wearing sunglasses. The sunglasses screened out ultraviolet light. Was it necessary for this part of the spectrum to be received not just by the skin, but through the eye? Was full-spectrum light essential for human health? Ott began to spend as much time as he could outside in natural light, without glasses of any kind, and his arthritis bothered him less and less. He was soon playing golf and walking without his cane.

John Ott has since founded the Environmental Health and Light Research Institute for the purpose of conducting research into the relationship of natural light to health and furthering the use of full-spectrum lighting in homes and other buildings and ultraviolet-transmitting glass in eyeglasses and windows.

There have been other findings that seem to indicate that Ott's conclusions are well-founded. Take the case of a group of

Cree Indians in Manitoba, for example. They had an exceptionally high rate of pterygium, an abnormal growth on the eyeball that eventually destroys sight. Investigation disclosed the fact that this group of people had been issued specially designed sunglasses in connection with an experiment set up to study problems of glare from snow and ice. The sunglasses were of the wraparound type and were fitted snugly to the head with leather padding to prevent any direct sunlight from reaching the eye. In other words, ultraviolet light was not hitting the eyes of these Indians.

In checking individuals who had become victims of pterygium while in the tropics on military duty, it was found that they, too, had all worn prescription sunglasses.

Obrig Laboratories, north of Sarasota, Florida, is a firm that manufactures contact lenses. During an epidemic in which 6,000 residents of Sarasota County were sick with the flu, not one employee of Obrig Laboratories fell victim to the flu bug. Is it just a coincidence that Obrig was the first concern to use full-spectrum lighting and ultraviolet-transmitting windowpanes?

One of the apostles of getting more sunlight into the home, Dr. Solco Tromp, feels it is desirable because of "the important physiological effects of natural light on a number of endocrine functions and the natural daily biological rhythms of man."

It is possible for you to buy ultraviolet-transmitting window glass and spectacles, and you can install full-spectrum lighting in your home. And, of course, you can spend as much time outdoors as possible. You don't have to be out in full sun. Open shade provides all the wavelengths of natural sunlight.

The Healing Power of Light

Scientific work on the health effects of sunlight has led to a medical breakthrough: phototherapy. Medicine is using artificial light given off by various kinds of electric lamps to treat a wide range of ailments, from psoriasis to brain tumors.

One of the most dramatic uses of the healing power of light is in saving the lives of newborn babies, particularly premature infants in whom red blood cells sometimes die and degenerate into a substance called bilirubin, causing the skin to look yellow. A properly functioning liver metabolizes bilirubin, but in some babies the liver does not begin to function fully for a few days. The result is that the bilirubin is not carried off as it should be. The situation can be dangerous because the bilirubin tends to become concentrated in certain parts of the brain, where it can cause severe damage, even death.

Medicine was long baffled by this condition. Then in 1958 an English physician, Dr. R. J. Cremer, working at General Hospital in Rockford, England, noticed something about the jaundiced babies in the hospital nursery. Those near the windows appeared to be less yellow than those in bassinets away from the windows. Was the light doing something to reduce the bilirubin? Lab tests seemed to confirm that it was.

In the United States, Dr. Jerold P. Lucey and his associates at the University of Vermont College of Medicine provided further proof. After exposing babies affected with the bilirubin syndrome to ordinary fluorescent lamps for three to four days, they found that the British researchers were right. In spite of the inadequately functioning livers of the infants, they were successfully excreting the bilirubin.

The precise ways in which light accomplishes this medical miracle has not been determined, but there is no question of its effectiveness. Exposure to light has become the standard treatment for bilirubin syndrome.

If you have any kind of an ailment that requires taking medication, either orally or by injection, you may soon be taking your medicine in a totally new way. It will go to work in your body through the help of sunlight falling on your skin! Sound fantastic? Not when you examine some amazing facts about skin now known to medical researchers. The human epidermis contains enzymes that have the capacity to metabolize certain substances touching it. The enzymatic action breaks down the substance and permits it to enter the bloodstream. However, what triggers their action is not just the substance on the skin. It's the *light striking the skin* that makes the otherwise inactive enzymes get busy doing their thing.

To utilize this phenomenon, medication could simply be applied, as a salve or powder, to a limited area—on the wrist, for instance. If the enzymes naturally in the skin were not of a type that would metabolize a particular drug, new enzymes could be introduced along with the medication.

"The skin," says Dr. David R. Bickers, Case Western Reserve University research dermatologist, "may be able to process drugs in ways otherwise difficult or impossible. It can render weak compounds more powerful, detoxify properties of others, minimizing side effects that occur in orally administered medications which must go through the gastrointestinal tract. Skin-absorbed drugs go directly into the bloodstream."

A light-research study conducted at MIT has led to a discovery of profound importance for anybody over the age of fifty, one offering a powerful argument for the benefits of retiring to a sunny climate. One of the problems that older people face is faulty utilization of calcium. Dr. Richard Wurtman and his associate, Robert Neer, set out to discover if light was a factor in enabling the body to make better use of calcium in the diet. In their initial experiment, the researchers worked with two groups of elderly men in the Chelsea Soldiers Home near Boston. After seven weeks of exposure to ordinary fluorescent lamps for three and a half hours a day, the men were found to absorb 40 percent of the calcium they ingested. For the next four weeks (two in February, two in March), one group remained under the same low-level lighting. For the same period, the other group spent eight hours a day under much brighter lighting.

The ability of the low-level lighting group to absorb calcium fell by 25 percent. In the group under the higher-level lighting, the calcium absorption increased by 15 percent, even though the amount of light they were exposed to was no greater than one would encounter outside in fifteen minutes of summer sunlight. The MIT doctors concluded that the problem of inadequate calcium absorption is at least exacerbated, if not created, by lack of sufficient light.

The research of the phototherapists seems to point increasingly to a conclusion that is already widely believed by non-medical people: living where you can get more exposure to the sun is better for your health.

7

Air Ions–New Health Discovery

Biometeorologists have only recently discovered why healthy people, at certain times and in certain places, experience favorable or unfavorable physical and psychological reactions—reactions that cannot be attributed to factors of temperature, humidity, atmospheric pressure, or air pollution. What is responsible for such reactions is molecules in the air called *air ions,* electrified particles that you inhale with every breath you take.

What's an air ion? Simply, an air ion comes into being when a gaseous molecule ejects an electron and this displaced electron attaches itself to an adjacent molecule. The molecule that loses the electron is, by virtue of its loss, positively charged and is called a *positive ion.* The molecule that picks up the free electron becomes negatively charged and is called a *negative ion.* In relatively clean country air, there are usually between 1,500 and 4,000 ions (both kinds combined) per cubic centimeter of air, and the ratio is usually one negative ion to two positive ones.

The Ion Depletion Menace

Man has always breathed air ions. However, in modern times, the advances of technology have not only upset the balance of ions, creating a preponderance of positive ions, but in many situations and locations have drastically reduced the total number of ions in the air.

The result is that many people, including those who live and work in air-conditioned buildings, ride in automobiles, and breathe polluted urban air, are now inhaling a different kind of air from that our ancestors took into their lungs.

Between 30 percent and 50 percent of the population is believed to be particularly sensitive to ion conditions. Many suffer severe physical disabilities from breathing air that is either depleted of ions or that has an abnormally high percentage of positive ions. The air you breathe much of the time may have ten positive ions to one negative one, instead of the "natural" two-to-one ratio. The result is that you may be suffering from "positive ion poisoning."

Dr. Felix Sulman, the noted Israeli biometeorologist and a leading pioneer in the study of air ions, gives a grim picture of some of the dire effects of positive-ion poisoning: ". . . dryness, burning and itching of the nose; nasal obstruction; headaches; dry, scratchy throat; difficulty in swallowing; dry lips; dizziness; difficulty in breathing; and itching of the eyes. Positive ion poisoning affects patients after surgery and those suffering from varicose veins, heart infarcts, cardiac insufficiency, and arterial occlusion. It provokes neurohormonal changes which may precipitate thromboembolism."

The evil consequences of pos-ion poisoning don't stop with physical effects. Many people who display no physical symptoms suffer from a wide range of mental maladies. They include an inability to concentrate, irritability, sexual inadequacy, anxiety, and depression. Pos-ions have been described as the "ultimate downers," the hidden cause of many mental and emotional ills that drive millions of people to use tranquilizers and other drugs.

Discoveries about Ions

How can breathing positively charged molecules have these effects on the human body? Although ion research had been conducted in Europe in the twenties and thirties, confirming that ions appeared to have biological effects, it was not until the late 1950s that an American scientist, Dr. Albert Kreuger, solved the mystery.

Oddly enough, the first American to become interested in ions was not a scientist at all, but a California businessman whose company manufactured electric heaters. When customers complained that the heaters created headaches and made some allergy sufferers wheeze, it was discovered that the heaters were producing an abundance of positive ions. Puzzled and disturbed, Wesley Hicks, the company's president, turned to Stanford University engineers for help. They soon found that by changing the particular circuitry used in the heaters the emission of the positive ions could be eliminated.

The matter might have stopped there, but for Hicks's inquiring mind. What was there about positive ions, he wondered, that caused them to produce the ill effects? Hicks consulted Dr. Krueger, then head of the Department of Bacteriology at the University of California at Berkeley. To Hicks's surprise, the eminent microbiologist and pathologist confessed that he knew nothing about air ions.

"Never heard of them," Krueger admitted. He was stunned by the realization that science had been ignoring an atmospheric component that could have a biological effect as great as that described by Hicks. When he looked up the literature on the subject, he found that European and Japanese scientists were much more aware of the phenomenon than their American colleagues. But nobody anywhere really knew just how air ions produced the responses they do.

After his talks with Hicks, Krueger had to find out more about what ions did and how they did it. So great was his fascination with the subject that he resigned as head of the department and devoted all his time to probing the ion mystery. In his two rooms on the campus at Berkeley (which later became the Air Ion Laboratory, with backing from the Office of Naval

Research), Dr. Krueger discovered just what air ions, positive and negative, do to the human body. His discoveries will affect the health of millions.

In his quest for the ion secret, the California researcher's procedure was to raise generations of mice in different ionized atmospheres, some rich in positive ions, others containing large numbers of negative ions. By studying thousands of mice, both alive and in the dissecting room, he discovered that the animals that were subjected to air laden with positive ions had abnormally high amounts of the neurohormone serotonin in their blood and brain cells.

This was a truly exciting discovery, for at that time the medical world was just beginning to become aware of the role serotonin plays in human reactions. Discovered in 1957, it was being hailed as "the mystery hormone." Hundreds of scientists were enthusiastically carrying out experiments and writing papers about serotonin. It had been identified as a substance released into the blood when a person is subjected to emotional stress, but nobody had linked serotonin to ions.

Then, in 1960, Dr. Krueger was able to point to positive ions as serotonin releasers that caused the body to overdo the production of this hormone. An excess of serotonin might, under some circumstances, be beneficial, but more often it resulted in the wide range of distressing symptoms we've already mentioned.

The ion-induced serotonin reaction appears to come about in this way: When positive ions are inhaled, they enter the red corpuscles of the blood, along with the ordinary oxygen molecules that add oxygen to the hemoglobin. The positive ions "attack" the blood platelets, and the body responds to this attack by stepping up the production of serotonin.

Negative ions have the opposite effect. They are serotonin suppressors. While positive ions reduce the amount of life-giving oxygen reaching the blood, negative ions tend to increase it. They influence the cilia, the tiny hairs in the breathing passages which, as they vibrate at some fifteen times a second, keep dust and pollutants out of the lungs. Studies show that while positive ions depress the action of the cilia, negative ions increase their action, making them more effective.

There is some evidence that ions influence the body through another mechanism. Nerve endings in the skin may serve as receptors which set up responses in the body similar to those arising from the breathing in of the ions. There may be a relationship between the ion-sensitive areas on the skin and the acupuncture points mapped out by practitioners of that ancient healing art.

Ion Culprits in the Weather

Where you live has much to do with how many beneficial negative ions you get to breathe—and how many harmful positive ones assail you. The total number of ions and the mixture of them vary greatly from one location to the next. Natural processes related to terrain, sunlight, the earth's radioactivity, cosmic radiation, weather, and air pollution all contribute to these variations.

Certain weather conditions create abnormally large percentages of positive ions. If you live in an area that has many thunderstorms, you'll get considerably more exposure to the troublesome pos-ions. When a storm approaches, the moving masses of air create friction, in effect rubbing against each other, and this friction generates positive ions. This accounts for the discomfort felt by many people before and during a storm.

Dr. Sulman reports: "Not only weather-sensitive patients but many others may also react to air electricity in an adverse way. Some—particularly elderly people—may experience difficulty in breathing; asthmatics wheeze; rheumatic sufferers feel their joints; and, in general, sleeplessness or insomnia, irritability and tension are there for the asking. Hair and skin have an 'electrical charge.' Migraine patients suffer from severe attacks of headache, with nausea, vomiting, and optical disturbances. Heart cases complain of palpitations, heart pain, and oppression. Women before the age of menopause complain of hot flushes with sweat or chills. Hay fever patients suffer attacks of rhinitis with conjunctivitis, though it is not their real hay fever season. Giddiness, tremor, and balance disturbances may appear, as well as diarrhea and a constant desire to urinate."

The most virulent weather-related onslaughts of positive ions come with the foehn winds, excessively warm winds that blow in many mountainous areas of the world. In the United States and Canada they occur in the mountain areas of the West, where they are called chinooks, and in the Southwest and California, where they bear the names "Santa Ana" and "California Norther."

In California the Northers are dreaded by inhabitants of the Sacramento Valley. In the Gold Rush days the effects of these winds on people were often cited as an extenuating circumstance in cases of mayhem and murder. It is said that "a Californian during a Norther drives as if convinced that every other man or woman behind the wheel is his mortal enemy." So notorious are the effects of the Santa Ana that the chamber of commerce of the community bearing that name once petitioned the state legislature for a name change. It was an affront to their fair community, they averred, to be known by the same name as that devilish phenomenon.

The chinook is less maligned. People who live in the Rocky Mountain West where it occurs are more willing to overlook its bad effects on people, since its warmth is often a welcome relief from the cold of winter. Known as the "snow eater," it often strips a foot or more of snow from the ground in a few hours, not melting it into water that will soak into the soil, but turning it into vapor in a process that meteorologists call "sublimation." On the ranges of the West, starving cattle standing in deep snow have often been saved as the quickly disappearing snow leaves grass exposed. Temperatures have been known to jump as much as forty degrees in a few minutes. In one case in Montana it went from −5° F. to 54° F.—a sixty-degree rise—in less than an hour.

Grateful as people might be on occasion for the warmth of the foehns, it has always been recognized that their influence on some individuals is disastrous. From the times of the early pioneers to the present, the records abound with observations such as, "Before and during a chinook I am troubled with the fidgets" . . . "You'd think I'd welcome them, but instead I become worried and depressed when the warm winds blow" . . . "The foehn gives me an awful headache, so bad I can hardly stand it."

Although physicians and meteorologists had always observed the dire effects of these "wicked winds" on people, the exact cause of the effects was a mystery which biometeorologists began to solve only in the 1960s. It had been thought that various physical and psychological manifestations were brought about by changes in pressure, humidity, and temperature, although it was difficult to explain why people experienced problems long before the troublesome winds began to blow.

The explanation turns out to be positive-ion poisoning, which induces the serotonin reaction. Once scientists recognized this, they had no trouble pinpointing the ion factor in the foehns and related winds. At various stages of the foehn phenomenon the total number of ions increased greatly, with a disproportionate increase in the number of positive ions. Israeli scientists, for example, found that some ten hours before the wind called the sharav started to blow, the number of ions jumped from 1,500 to 2,600 per cubic centimeter. The most significant change occurred in ion balance. The ratio of positive to negative ions soared from its basic 2-to-1 to 33-to-1.

The Air Pollution Factor

No natural factor of geography or weather creates such a plague of positive ions as does the air pollution of urban areas. In our cities the total number of ions is drastically reduced, and a preponderance of ions present are positive ones. As we said earlier, country air contains from 1,500 to 4,000 ions per cubic centimeter. Near a busy freeway the count can drop to 500. On a congested city street there may be as few as 200. Other factors conspire to reduce the number of negative ions. Negative ions tend to join with pollution particles, causing them to become larger and heavier until they finally fall to the ground. Automobiles do more than their share of the dirty work, not only by spewing pollutants into the air, but just by moving. Cars act as negative-ion destroyers because as they move, they become positively charged. This results in their attracting negative ions and repelling positive ones. Thus heavy traffic has the effect of removing the good ions from the air.

Unfortunately, as with other forms of air pollution, there's no escape indoors. In fact, the air in your home, office, or other place of work may be even worse, in terms of ionization, than the air outdoors. Air passing over metal, as it does in the ducts of heating and air-conditioning systems, actually produces positive ions. And the surviving negative ions that do manage to get into the air of your heated or air-conditioned rooms suffer a further diminishment. Synthetic fabrics have a positive charge and therefore attract negative ions, drawing them out of the air. The very clothing you wear, the upholstered furniture you sit on, the carpets you walk on are all taking their toll of negative ions and therefore damaging the air you breathe.

The Geography of the Good Ions

Where can you find more negative ions and what can they do for you? As you have already read, there are a lot more of them in rural locations than there are in urban areas. In country air there are roughly 700 to 1,300 negative ions per cubic centimeter of air entering your lungs, at the natural ratio of one negative ion to two positive ones. This quantity of negatives is certainly enough to offset any ill effects the positives may have.

We should emphasize that positive ions are not in themselves harmful. It's only when there are too few ions of either kind, such as in the "dead" air of city streets or in certain heated or air-conditioned buildings, or when the proportion of positive ions to negative ones is very high, that they do their harm.

There are certain geographical locations where you'll find vastly more negative ions than in the normal country air we've referred to. One location is the seashore, where ocean waves dashing against the shore send up spray that is loaded with negative ions. This is why most of us find a particular exhilaration in walking on a beach or clambering about on a rock-bound coast.

The perfect place to live—from an ion standpoint—would be next to a waterfall, for falling water produces a tremendous number of ions, with a preponderance of negative ions. The ion count in close proximity to a small waterfall can be astonishingly high. As many as 200,000 ions per cubic centimeter have been recorded within a few yards of falling water. A large waterfall, such as the often photographed one in Yosemite National Park, can produce enough ions to affect the entire Yosemite Valley. Measurements at Niagara Falls have not, to our knowledge, been extensively made, but it is believed that both Niagara Falls, New York, and Niagara Falls, Ontario, are blessed with unusually high numbers of air ions. It has even been suggested that this may be the reason the Falls have been such a favored spot for honeymooners.

Unfortunately, very few people can live near a waterfall. More, of course, might be able to live near a rushing stream, which is also a good ion producer. More still might manage to move to the mountains, another favored place for ion production. Many conditions in mountainous regions—the evergreens, the intensity of the sunlight, and the greater radioactivity of the rocks and soil—contribute to the generation of large quantities of ions. (The radioactivity is nothing to be feared. There is a certain amount of natural background radiation everywhere, all at a low level that mankind has always lived with comfortably on this planet.)

How to Get More Healthful Ions into Your Life

We are not dependent on nature to provide us with beneficial quantities of negative ions. Engineers have devised various machines that produce them. Most are simple devices that plug into an electrical outlet. Smaller versions can even be plugged into the dashboard of a car. In Europe, Israel, and Japan they are made by a number of manufacturers and sold in appliance stores. In the Soviet Union, a do-it-yourself kit is offered with readily assembled components.

In the United States during the late fifties and early sixties, several American companies started making the machines. However, they made wild and unproved statements, claiming their devices could cure many ills. This brought about a Food and Drug Administration ban on advertising negative-ion machines as having medical uses; they could be billed only as "air cleaners." They are still made by a few American companies, but are not much advertised. Lifting of the FDA ban on advertising their therapeutic value will probably have to await the results of much more research in this pioneering field. Machines for professional use are available and are used by a number of American researchers. They have also been studied by various government agencies, including NASA and the Office of Naval Research.

It is not within the scope of this book to go into all the medical uses of negative-ion therapy. It is widely used in many European countries for the treatment of a variety of diseases, most of them respiratory. In this country, negative ions, until now, have not commonly been used in medical practice. However, tests have been conducted with impressive results. For instance, Dr. A. P. Wehner treated patients for emphysema, bronchitis, and various nasal and sinus conditions of allergic origin with negative-ionized air at his clinic in Dallas. Of the 1,000 patients covered in one of his reports, 42.3 percent experienced significant improvement and 20 percent some improvement from twice-daily half-hour sessions of breathing negative-ionized air over a period of twenty to thirty days. At the University of

Pennsylvania Graduate Hospital, Dr. Igho Kornblueh used negative ions to treat patients suffering from bronchial asthma and cited 63-percent success. It was reported that "they come in sneezing, eyes watering, noses itching, worn out from lack of sleep, so miserable they can hardly walk. Fifteen minutes in front of the negative-ion machine and they feel so much better they don't want to leave."

The greatest potential for the power of negative ions probably lies not in the treatment of disease, but in their potential benefit to healthy individuals. A distinguished Russian physician, A. L. Tchijewsky, points out: "Negatively ionized air . . . can be used for increasing physical work capacity and improving the general tone of healthy people." Dr. Krueger agrees, stating that "work capacity, general health, and tranquillity are improved by exposure to high concentrations of negative ions."

Should you try a negative-ion machine? Some people are astonished by the beneficial results, others say they feel no difference. Since it's such a highly personal matter, you would have to experiment before you knew what such a machine would do for you. You can be sure of one thing anyway: in thousands of tests by medical researchers, negative ions have never been known to hurt anybody. Ill or healthy, young or old, you're perfectly safe in trying a negative-ion generator. They are customarily sold on a trial basis, since it's generally recognized that not everybody benefits. However, don't expect to get any medical advice about the use of such a machine.

Paradoxically, negative ions not only give you more energy; they can also induce sleep. There is evidence that serotonin levels build up in some people during sleep, causing them to sleep poorly. A lot of people sleep better, therefore, in a room equipped with a negative-ion generator. A doctor we know reports that he had a patient who suffered from insomnia and was worried, as was the doctor, about becoming dependent on sleeping pills. After he acquired a negative-ion generator for his bedroom he never had any trouble sleeping.

If you'd like to be breathing more negative ions, but don't

want to get a negative-ion machine and can't consider moving to the mountains or the seashore, it's good to know that you have a negative-ion producer in your home right now: the bathroom shower. It generates negative ions in quantities, especially if set on a fine spray. This is probably one of the reasons showers are so refreshing. It isn't just the pleasant sensation of the water on your body. Actually, any running water generates some negative ions. Even a flushing toilet releases a brief burst of them.

Growing plants in your home or office helps, too. They create ions, as do trees in your yard, particularly evergreens.

To cut down on the destruction of negative ions in your home, you can tear out the nylon carpeting, get rid of the plastic-covered chairs and the synthetic-fabric draperies. By using natural materials—wood or brick floors, cottons and wools for drapes and rugs—you can make your home a considerably more comfortable place in which to live. We speak from experience, for we did all these things and we at least *feel* as though we've benefited. You can also change your way of dressing. Stop wearing synthetic fabrics and switch to garments made of natural fibers. You might end up agreeing with those people who claim they have been revitalized by negative ions, even going so far as to say that the electrified particles have helped their sex lives.

8

Are High Altitudes More Healthful?

In recent years, many Americans, seeking that "better place to live," have moved to the mountain West. The populations of Denver and Albuquerque, as well as many high-altitude smaller cities, have soared. Most surveys indicate that the influx of newcomers will continue, at an accelerated pace, in the years ahead.

Judging by the vast number of inquiries to western chambers of commerce, great numbers of vacationers, skiers, college students, and retirees, impressed by what they've heard or read or what they've seen on their own visits to the mountain states, would like to move to the high country of Arizona, New Mexico, Colorado, Nevada, Utah, Wyoming, Idaho, or Montana.

Why does high-altitude living appeal to so many people? It's a combination of many things. Some people who want to move to the mountain West aren't even thinking much about the altitude; they're dreaming of all that space, the vast areas of wilderness, the spectacular scenery, the varied recreational opportunities, or of just "getting away from it all." But there are many who are thinking about climate—what it might do for their comfort and their health.

For hundreds of years, all over the world, doctors have sent their patients to high mountain retreats where they were expected to recover from a wide variety of ills. Before the 1880s, Colorado, with its high altitude, bracing air, and mineral springs, had become a Mecca for invalids hoping to recover their health. One of the earliest consumptives to settle in the Denver area was Andrew Sagendorf. He was carried there in a wagon, along with the boards to build a coffin for him should such action prove necessary on the way. He spent the next fifty-four years helping to build Denver.

The tales are legion and the list of health seekers is a long one. F. O. Stanley, for instance, was sent to Colorado in 1903 in hopes that it would prolong his life for "a year or so." He lived for thirty-seven more years, not dying until his ninety-fourth year. During that time he invented the Stanley Steamer motorcar. And there was John B. Stetson, who left Philadelphia in ill health and camped out in the Pikes Peak region, where he found his health restored. He lived to design that famous western hat that bears his name.

Many of Colorado's health seekers were doctors. Charles Denison, who moved west from Connecticut, regained his health after a short residence. He was one of the first physicians to recognize the need for a formal, systematic study of the relationship of climate to disease and was one of the founders of the American Climatological Association. In Denison's time most of the sick migrants who came to the high-altitude west were victims of tuberculosis, but Denison was quick to see that the mountain climate also helped people suffering from a wide range of respiratory and rheumatoid ailments. Many of today's newcomers to high-altitude areas are victims of asthma, allergies, and arthritis who are finding improved health in new homes high above sea level.

High-Country Climates

Mountains, of course, catch clouds, but in the mountain West the clouds are usually of the quickly passing variety, so the sun shines a large percentage of the time. Denver and Albuquerque, for instance, get 70 to 80 percent of possible winter sunshine, while cities like Buffalo and Detroit get barely 30 percent. High altitude also affects the quality of sunlight. The thinner atmosphere absorbs less of the sun's radiation; the higher you go, the more intense the sunlight. Air temperature can be down around the freezing point and yet your skin, if exposed to the sun in a wind-free location, will feel comfortably warm. High-altitude sunlight also has a greater amount of ultraviolet in it, since not as much of the UV is screened out by the atmosphere.

The mountain states of the West have low humidities. The cold of winter is a "dry cold," and the heat of summer vanishes every evening. In the summertime in Denver, for instance, there is often a difference of thirty degrees or more between the daytime high and the nighttime low. Summer nights in high-altitude places are always cool. The thinner air quickly gives up its heat.

There is also a meteorological phenomenon arising from the very presence of the mountains. As soon as the sun goes down, the cooler air at higher elevations begins to flow downhill into the valleys, where most mountain-area communities are situated. This creates a cool breeze, the arrival of which can, in some locations, be predicted almost to the minute.

There's also a special quality to high-altitude air, best described as "invigorating." Some biometeorologists believe it is caused by the presence of large amounts of negative ions. Though this has yet to be proved, it is possible that the ions are just one of many factors that make high-altitude climates exhilarating and relaxing at the same time.

Not everybody likes a mountain climate. The complaint we've heard most often, usually from new arrivals, is that mountain weather is too volatile. You no sooner get adjusted to one kind of weather than another kind comes along and takes its place. There are often sudden, dramatic shifts of temperature, sunshine, clouds, winds, and precipitation factors. However, weather changes in mountain areas are often very localized and are not brought about by large air movements.

Some mountain areas are windy, particularly certain locations in valleys or at the mouths of canyons. There are also special mountain winds, like the foehn, that trouble many people. Biometeorologists attribute this wind's evil effects to the fact that it is drying and has a high content of positive ions, triggering the physiological responses described in the previous chapter. However, foehn winds do not occur often, nor do they blow in all mountain locations.

What Altitude Does to You

A discussion of the physiological effects of high altitude really must begin with an answer to the question, "How high is high?" Dr. C. B. Favour, noted medical researcher at the National Jewish Hospital in Denver, points out that "to a sea-level lubber, Denver's lofty mile-high altitude seems very high. To the physiologist, however, Denver is just barely high enough to be called high altitude."

For our purposes, the altitude of Denver and Albuquerque is "high." We define any community of 4,000 feet or over as high because beginning at that altitude, many people notice some difference in the way they feel.

When we say that the air is "thinner" at high altitudes, we mean that the atmospheric pressure is less and that air molecules are farther apart. At high altitudes you have to breathe in more air to provide your body with the oxygen it needs. This explains why high-altitude dwellers have greater lung capacity and why racehorses and sometimes athletes are trained at high-altitude locations.

You must take in half a pint of oxygen per minute just to keep yourself alive, at complete rest. An office worker or a person doing light physical work needs a pint per minute. Average weekend recreational activity can double, triple, or even quadruple your requirement to as much as two quarts. Strenuous activity, such as tennis or cross-country skiing, can push bodily needs up to six quarts per minute.

You need these amounts of oxygen wherever you are—at sea level or at 20,000 feet. At higher altitudes you must breathe more rapidly, more deeply, or both, in order to get the required amount of oxygen from the thinner air.

At altitudes under 4,000 feet you're unlikely to notice any difference in your breathing, but at some point in altitudes above that level you will begin to notice a difference. There is a great variation in individual reactions. Some people observe a change in their breathing rate at about 5,000 feet; others notice no change at all at 8,000 feet. Of course, there *is* a difference; we're talking about *awareness* of the difference.

Is the kind of breathing required at high altitudes good or bad for your health? In general, medical authorities say, it's good. It strengthens the heart and lungs. To get the necessary amount of oxygen into the system at high altitudes the body produces more oxygen-carrying red blood cells. Studies show that a person coming from a low altitude is, within two hours of arrival at Denver's altitude, already beginning to produce more such cells.

A few people do show some ill effects upon first coming to high altitude. Dr. Favour says of new arrivals in Denver, "Some who have busy schedules may experience more yawning and tiredness during the daylight hours, a tendency to insomnia, thirst, and unusual breathlessness on exertion, such as carrying suitcases or climbing stairs. . . . Within a few days the newcomer brightens up and is his usual self. The same thing can happen to a Denverite who goes to an even higher altitude of 8,000 to 10,000 feet. Lowlanders going to this level will experience more marked effects. Tiredness, headaches, and active kidneys are not uncommon."

Probably more questions are asked about what altitude does to one's heart than about any other physical effect of coming to the high country. The answers given by medical doctors are reassuring. High altitudes can cause some people's hearts to speed up, but very little else happens to a healthy heart at high altitudes. (We're not talking about very high altitudes, or climbing difficult mountains.)

Does High-Altitude Living Lengthen Life?

What about those high-altitude dwellers you've read about who live to such ripe old ages? It's long been known that inhabitants of the Andes, for instance, have a much lower death rate from heart disease than do residents of the United States. In the forty-five-to-sixty-four age group, the death rate per 100,000 from arteriosclerosis in the United States in a ten-year period was 389.5. Among Peruvians living at above 10,000 feet the rate was only 41.6—about one-tenth of the U.S. rate. The death rate in the United States from hypertensive heart diseases was 61.3; in Peru it was only 15.8.

The significance of these statistics is more evident in the context of the study made in the United States by doctors from Harvard, Case Western Reserve, and the University of New Mexico medical schools. Their medical investigation, carried out in New Mexico, clearly established the fact that there is a direct relationship between high-altitude living and heart-disease death rate, at least among males. (The relationship is not marked among females.)

In a project extending over a fifteen-year period, the researchers, Drs. Edward Mortimer, Jr., Richard R. Monson, and Brian MacMahon, concluded that altitudes of 5,000 feet and up reduce the rate of heart-disease deaths, with the most pronounced decrease of all occurring in men living at altitudes of over 7,000 feet. In fact, the death rate at this altitude was 28 percent less than that for men at a 3,000-foot altitude.

The doctors were able to eliminate factors other than altitude that might account for the striking differences. Ethnic background? The low-altitude population had about the same mix as that in the high altitudes. Drinking water? In the case of New Mexico this factor was ruled out because at the lower altitudes hard water was as prevalent as at the higher ones (as you will read in Chapter 11, the softer the water, the higher the incidence of heart disease). Were lower-altitude people smoking more? A study of cigarette sales tax receipts indicated there was no detectable difference in the smoking habits of the two groups.

The researchers have not reached a firm conclusion as to just how high altitude lengthens lives. However, they point out a number of known facts. Living at high altitude "deters the development of hypertension. Blood pressure, particularly systolic, is lower at high altitude, and sequential changes with age are less pronounced than at sea level. A second effect of high altitude that might exert a protective influence is increased myocardial vascularity."

According to the report, the most important factor is that the heart works harder at high altitudes and therefore is made stronger. Normal, everyday work activities at high altitudes give the heart the kind of workout it gets only from more strenuous activity at sea level.

9

Sex, Procreation, and the Weather

Do weather and climate really have anything to do with sex and procreation? Are there seasons of peak sexual activity that correspond to the seasons of the year? Are there times of the year in which it's better to be born?

The answers, in order, are: "Definitely yes," "Probably yes," and "Maybe yes."

For all the vast amount of sexual research that has been done in recent years—Kinsey, Masters and Johnson, et al.—no medical researchers have as yet confined themselves to a study of sex as it relates to climate, weather, and the environment.

However, some researches conducted in related areas suggest that your sex drives, fertility, and even the sex and intelligence of your offspring are influenced by ups and downs of the barometer, temperature, the kind and number of ions in the air, the season of the year, and the place where you live.

Current sex research has at least put to rest the popular myth that women in the tropics mature earlier than women in temperate climates. Marriage follows so soon after first menstruation in the tropics that eighteenth- and nineteenth-century explorers and missionaries, seeing mothers who were sixteen, fifteen, or even younger, just assumed that they matured earlier sexually. In more developed countries, the onset of menstruation and the arrival of the first offspring do not follow in rapid sequence.

It is an interesting fact that today, in the more artificial climates of our urban areas, city girls, on the average, mature about half a year earlier than rural girls.

Aphrodisiacs in the Weather

Is there something in the weather that can increase sex drive? Yes, say Drs. Richard Udry and Naomi Morris, of the Institute for Sex Research at the University of Indiana. They made an extensive study of the sexual activities of volunteers from that region and discovered that the "coital calendars" of women followed a definite seasonal pattern. They reported a much higher rate of intercourse during the summer months. The peak came in July, between the twenty-sixth and thirty-first weeks of the year, with a frequency rate 10 percent higher than that of the annual average.

This observation checks with the findings of a research program carried out by Canadian scientists, who discovered that sex drive among the males they studied was highest in midsummer, lowest in midwinter.

Before either of these studies was made, Dr. Clarence Mills, the University of Cincinnati biometeorologist, concluded that extremes of outside temperature, no matter what the heating or cooling conditions were inside, tended to inhibit sexual drive.

Storms are a specific weather phenomenon that various researchers think may have an influence on the libido. "I don't know whether sexual desires could be said to go up and down with the barometer," Dr. William Petersen once remarked to one of the authors of this book, "but I've known of people who were sexually depressed when the pressure began to drop a day or two before the actual arrival of the front. These same people were stimulated when the storm had passed and the barometer was rising."

In an informal survey, we found many people who were convinced that storms were influential, but we couldn't find any consistent pattern to their reactions. "I find thunderstorms stimulating. There's an excitement to them. Must be the electricity in the air or something" . . . "Excited by storms? Quite the contrary. They're frightening and disturbing to me. I just feel irritable" . . . "Well, storm conditions make me feel more energetic in general, and of course that might increase sex drive."

The consensus among biometeorologists we talked to is that weather changes can increase the flow of adrenaline and step up metabolism and the delivery of oxygen to the bodily tissues, including, therefore, those of the sexual organs. One M.D., though he did not know of any medical study that bore out the view, felt that there could well be an increase in the bodily levels of the male hormone, testosterone.

Some studies indicate that heat and accompanying high humidity act as depressants to sexual activity. However, researchers in the Human Sexuality Program of the Albert Einstein College of Medicine in New York point out that this may not be a specific sexual effect. Heat causes bodily energy in general to drop, so a lowering of sex drives may be simply a result of the general physical condition. All investigators in the field throw up their hands about the possibility of getting really definite answers about weather effects in an age of air conditioning.

"It must be noted," one researcher told us, "that we probably never will find a temperature condition that's a universal turn-on. Some like it hot—some like it cold, and some . . ."

Light—Sex Trigger?

Dr. Alfred Kinsey, the pioneer sex researcher, did not, in his history-making investigations, make much of an inquiry into the subject of how weather affects either sexual desire or sexual performance, but from casual comments gathered in his surveys he drew the conclusion that good weather stimulated sexual activity. He thought that being out in the sunshine helped, but saw that as part of a total pattern. The best aphrodisiacs, he felt, are fresh air, sunshine, exercise, good food, and adequate sleep.

Light may be a key factor in triggering various sexual responses. Numerous lab experiments with animals have shown that it has a marked effect. Dr. Richard Wurtman, the MIT endocrinologist, reports that when he kept rats under fluorescent lighting, gonad growth was retarded. Rats kept under lamps that delivered a full spectrum of light, like that of sunlight, had sex glands that grew at a normal rate. Many other animal experiments by biological researchers, using mice, rats, hamsters, and birds, have confirmed these findings.

Anthropologists, who have observed human beings in all parts of the world, report that light definitely affects the human reproductive system. Eskimo women, they point out, do not menstruate during the months of darkness. When they receive no sunlight, they become unfertile. It has also been observed that there is a drop in sexual drive among Eskimos during these same winter months, but not on account of a lack of warm sleeping quarters. Eskimo dwellings, including the igloo, are kept at high temperatures. The inquisitive anthropologist Vilhjalmur Stefansson once took readings in igloos of a tribe deep in the Arctic circle and found that 90° F. was not an uncommon temperature inside these ice houses.

Dr. Joseph Meites, a Michigan State researcher, reports, "In the spring a young squirrel's fancy turns because the days are getting longer, and exposure to longer light periods sets off a chain reaction involving the brain and pituitary gland, resulting in releases of hormones that affect sex hormone levels and in turn cause the sex glands to enlarge."

The bodily mechanism that responds to light and by doing so touches off human sexual reactions is thought to be the pineal gland, that mysterious pea-sized organ at the base of the brain which has often been called the "third eye." It is known that the pineal gland is affected by several different wavelengths of visible light.

One biometeorologist told us that he believed the little-known hormone norepinephrine to be worth some serious speculation. It is a hormone similar to adrenaline in its effects and is stored in cells located in the nerve endings of the body.

"We've found," he said, "that the pineal gland contains a lot of norepinephrine. Personally, I think it's an active substance—maybe *the* active substance—in sex arousal. We have already demonstrated that it has a lot to do with general functioning, how alert you are, how active. Of course, it's all tied in with other endocrinological systems, but I'm convinced that an important direction to take in future research is to explore the relationship of norepinephrine to sexual drive."

The mysterious effects of light may account for the fact that many people—males in particular—who have moved to a warmer climate, and therefore spend more time outdoors in the sunshine, report that their sex lives experience an unexpected revival.

A sixty-two-year-old engineer who retired to Florida happily reports: "I'd begun to fear that I wasn't going to have much of a sex life anymore, but when we got settled here, I found myself sexually active again. Well, not every night, of course, but at least once, maybe twice, a week. Phenomenal. Climate? Who knows? But I am living a very different kind of life—getting outdoors every day—jogging—riding an exercycle between times. I feel I'm in better physical shape than I've been in years."

Of course, it's safe to say that the improved sexual life of this particular individual was a result of many factors of more healthful living. However, there's a real possibility that sunlight was playing the major role. His whole endocrinological system may have been stimulated in a way it hadn't been in years.

One of the questions we've asked hundreds of Sunbelt retirees is, "Has your sex life improved?" Many didn't want to answer at all, but many volunteered that there had been a marked change for the better. We observed that the retirees who had moved to warmer climates and who were leading more active lives (many in their sixties, even seventies, had taken up hiking, jogging, swimming, even tennis) reported that their sex lives had been rejuvenated after they started such regimens.

Significant? We think it is, and a number of M.D.'s and bio-meteorologists with whom we discussed the matter agreed with us. Whether it all has a physiological or psychological basis, whether it is endocrinological or metabolic or related to sunlight or weather, it seems, in the words of one midwestern physician, "worthy of a lot of thought, and is probably a good recommendation for a change of climate, particularly if it brings with it a change in life-style and physical activity."

The Sex Powers of Negative Ions

Do ions in the air affect your sex life? Yes, say many medical researchers. These electrified particles may be acting as turn-ons or turn-offs. Negative ions, the "good" kind, may be one of the keys to a vigorous sex life, and positive ions, the "bad" kind, so ubiquitous in our urban world, may account for many of the sexual problems that are also ubiquitous.

The possible detrimental effects of positive ions on sexual functioning have been traced by Dr. Felix Sulman to their role in producing the hormone serotonin. In a classic study he was able to determine that positive ions create reactions in the female reproductive system. To twenty women desiring legal abortions, Dr. Sulman gave a drug (since banned in Israel) that produces quantities of serotonin. All of the women aborted. Later the Israeli researcher administered a serotonin-reducing drug to 100 women who had histories of miscarriages. None of these women had succeeded in carrying a baby to full term. With the serotonin eliminated, almost all of them went to full-term pregnancies.

From this experiment Dr. Sulman and other scientists deduce the ill effects of positive ions in the air. Since serotonin has been demonstrated to have such a potent effect on reproduction, and since serotonin is produced in the body by a high proportion of positive ions in the air, it seems reasonable to assume that air ions might have effects that extend to all aspects of sexuality.

There are many reports in the medical literature of sexual

disabilities occurring when weather conditions produce large amounts of positive ions—particularly when "ill winds" like the foehn, the sharav, and the Santa Ana are blowing. A California doctor says he has established a definite relationship between temporary drops in sexual drive and the Santa Ana wind. Dr. Sulman's studies of the sharav have indicated a widespread drop in sexual activities during the onslaught of that drying, positive-ion-laden wind.

The demonstrated potency of negative ions in stepping up sexual drive is one more benefit they offer. Many of the experiments carried out by Dr. Albert Kreuger in his Air Ions Laboratory at the University of California have produced striking evidence that organisms of all kinds are affected by negative ions. In one of his tests Dr. Kreuger raised silkworms in atmospheres enriched with negative ions. He found that the larvae matured earlier and that the adults mated earlier and produced much more luxuriant cocoons. This discovery has been put to work by the operators of Japanese silk farms, who use negative-ion generators to make their silkworms more productive.

A report of research carried out at the University of Milan notes an increase in sexual activity as a result of exposure to air ions. In a series of animal experiments the testicles and ovaries of animals exposed to high concentrations of negative ions for ninety-six hours showed a definite stimulation of the maturation of a large number of cells.

Is the secret of Niagara Falls's longtime popularity as a honeymoon spot the presence of the large numbers of negative ions generated by the Falls? We know a young couple who repeatedly go back to camp beside their "favorite waterfall," one in southern Colorado. They first discovered it years ago when, tired from a long day's hike, they unexpectedly came upon the falls. It was sending out a misty spray over a large area. "Our fatigue just vanished," they told us. "We felt an electrifying sense of exhilaration. We decided to camp there that night, and . . . well . . . wow!"

Many similar reports come from people who have installed negative-ion generators in their bedrooms. "It transformed our marriage," one European enthusiast avers.

Imagination or ions? "It doesn't make all that much difference, does it?" a noted sex researcher asks. "I can only say that the machines have made a difference for a lot of people. But whether it's the ions or the belief in them I don't really know, or care. All sexual relations have such a large component of imagination anyway. A belief in an ion machine may be as good a fantasy as any."

The Season of Birth

Can the month in which a child is conceived have anything to do with determining its sex? Some researchers think that time of year, or at least the weather, has a lot to do with sex determination. Dr. William Petersen, who made a study of births in the Chicago area, found that babies conceived in December were statistically more likely to be boys. His explanation was that there was an increase in the metabolism of the ovum at fertilization, "producing a slight tendency toward maleness." This explanation is not widely accepted. Dr. Solco Tromp, for example, offered the theory that "shortly after fertilization" more cells of one sex or the other die and that cold-weather conception favored the survival of more male cells. Other researchers think that while the number of male conceptions in winter months is greater, the difference is so small as to be statistically insignificant or "confused" by other factors.

A Czechoslovakian medical scientist, Dr. Eugen Jonas, has achieved international fame (some would say notoriety) from his contention that the phases of the moon have more to do with determining the sex of offspring than seasons or weather or climate. Jonas's theory is based on studies of artificial insemination in which it has been observed that when a weak electric current is passed through a semen sample, male and female spermatozoa tend to be separated. The moon, of course, does affect the earth's magnetic field. This alteration, says Jonas, occurs as a result of the different positions of the moon. Using complicated calculations, he claims to have been 95 percent successful in predicting the sex of children born to 100 women who accepted his advice as to the time of conception to produce an offspring of the desired sex.

Some of the most intriguing biometeorological studies of sex and reproduction were made long ago by the tireless MIT researcher Ellsworth Huntington. After examining statistics concerning more than a million people he wrote a pioneering book, *Season of Birth*. Half a century after its publication it still challenges today's biometeorologists. Their researches tend to confirm his fascinating conclusions about the relation between the season of conception and the sex, intelligence, and health of children.

One of his conclusions was that children conceived in May and June get the best physical start in life. In a study of 6,500 people—3,500 conceived in June and born in February and March, 3,000 conceived in October and born in June or July— he found that those with June conception lived an average of 3.8 years longer than those conceived in October. Subsequent biometeorological studies have come up with somewhat different statistics, but all have had the same general results as the original Huntington findings.

Perhaps the most argued-about conclusion is that the season of conception has an effect on intelligence. Huntington's approach was to examine the birth dates of 80,000 people who had achieved prominence in their fields—doctors, lawyers, clergymen, scientists, authors, college professors, industrialists, and others listed in *Who's Who*. The MIT researcher concluded that the same rule he had established for general health and its resultant longevity also applied to intelligence. Recent research in the United States and Europe seems to confirm the finding that a disproportionate number of high achievers are born in February. However, this conclusion is contested by many medical authorities.

Biometeorologists also find solid evidence of seasonal influences at work in the conception of mentally retarded children. A landmark study by Drs. Hilda Knobloch and Benjamin Passamanik, of the Columbus Psychiatric Institute in Columbus, Ohio, reviewed the birth dates of mentally deficient children institutionalized over a thirty-five-year period. They found that an abnormally large number of schizophrenics were born in January and February, indicating that the very months of conception which seem to result in higher intelligence also result in more mental disturbances of a damaging nature.

It was also found that babies whose early fetal development happened to be taking place during very hot summers had a slightly greater chance of being mentally defective. One explanation for this is based on the fact that the third month after conception is the period during which the cerebral cortex of the fetus is organized. The mother's nutritional practices during that period are of crucial importance. Hot weather tends to reduce appetite and make people, even pregnant women, careless about what they eat. It has been demonstrated that if an expectant mother's protein intake is not as high as it should be during that period of gestation, the development of certain brain functions of the fetus may be inhibited.

Most biometeorologists and doctors tend to underplay the relation between season of birth and the child's health and mental capacity. Even those who do grant that there may be differences in children conceived at different times of the year argue that the mix of genetic and environmental factors is so complex that it is difficult to assess the significance of any single influence.

Medical knowledge in this field is not much greater than it was when Huntington published *Season of Birth*. At the time, the *Journal of the American Medical Association* commented, "This remarkable book is one of fundamental importance in human biology and should be read by every physician." But there it stands to this day—something to be read and talked about, perhaps, but, unfortunately, little more. Not many medical researchers have followed up on Huntington's findings.

Huntington himself remained convinced that parents could bequeath a child a legacy of health, and possibly greater intelligence, by arranging the time of conception. His final comment: "The extra years of life would not be added to the period of immaturity or to the period of decay in old age. Each of those would be shortened rather than lengthened by a widespread improvement in constitutional vigor. Thus the working period of life would be increased by perhaps five percent while the percentage of people too old and infirm to work would not show any corresponding increase. Moreover, during their working years people would enjoy better health than they do now. Hence they would lose less time in illness, do their work better, and behave more sanely because they would be less disturbed by the many minor ailments which do so much to warp our judgment and make us hard to get along with."

Will your child actually be more intelligent and healthier if conception occurs in the months of May or June? Should you plan it that way, as Huntington advised?

"Why not?" was the response of one obstetrician we consulted. "There just may be something to it."

10

Is Your Air
Fit to
Breathe?

Is air pollution all that bad? Aren't we all managing to survive, even though we're filling our lungs with poisons?

The answer to the first question: Yes, it *is* all that bad. In fact, it's probably worse than anyone really wants to think. And the answer to the second: A lot of us aren't surviving at all—and a great many more of us are just barely doing so.

As self-appointed searchers for better, more healthful places to live, we ask a third question: Is there any way you can escape the evil effects of air pollution? Later in this chapter we'll try to give some answers to that payoff question.

Air Pollution and Your Health

Just what do the pollutants in the air you breathe do to you? The American Lung Association, in its *Air Pollution Primer*, outlines the basic mechanisms: "Certain irritants, either gaseous or particulate, can slow down and even stop the action of the cilia and thus leave the sensitive underlying cells without protection. (The cilia are hair-like cells that line the airways. By their sweeping movement they propel the mucus—and the germs and dirt caught in it—out of the respiratory tract.) The irritants can cause the production of increased or thickened mucus. They can cause a constriction of the airways. They can induce swelling or excessive growth of the cells that form the lining of the airways. They can cause a loss of cilia or even of several layers of cells. Because of one or more of these reactions, breathing may become more difficult, and foreign matter, including bacteria and other microorganisms, may not be effectively removed."

Serious pulmonary disorders can be the result. The American Lung Association reports that deaths from emphysema and bronchitis double every five years in the United States and attributes much of this dramatic increase to the effects of air pollution on smokers and nonsmokers alike.

According to Dr. Russell Sherwin, Hastings Professor of Pathology at the University of Southern California, "It is not a question of *whether* a person has emphysema; it is just a question of *when* it becomes clinically significant. I believe everyone over twelve has emphysema. I know I can't find a normal lung in anyone over that age."

In a study by Drs. Lester Lave and Eugene Seskin, *Air Pollution and Human Health,* published by Johns Hopkins University Press, the noted scientists analyzed medical records in 100 American cities. They reached the conclusion that "air pollution does not simply 'harvest' deaths of susceptible individuals, but seems to reduce life expectancy in general." They calculate that if just the sulfur oxides in the air we breathe were cut by 50 percent, the nation's "death rate would drop an astonishing 4.7 percent."

In the Los Angeles and San Francisco areas, where lung cancer rates are more than double the national average, "the growing cancer rates correspond to growing air pollution levels," according to an official of California's Air Resources Board. This does not mean that California has the most polluted air in the nation. Many other areas have air that is just as bad, or even worse, but they do not experience the thermal inversion layer phenomenon, in which the polluted air is trapped down at the levels where people are forced to breathe it.

Is Your Air Fit to Breathe? 99

Short of killing us, air pollution makes an awful lot of us sick and miserable. Some physicians have defined what they call "air-pollution syndrome." One of the pioneers in setting up such a definition is Dr. Albert A. La Verne, who is associated with New York's Bellevue Hospital. This distinguished editor of *Physician's Drug Manual,* in his efforts to describe such a syndrome, carried out a study that turned up the following symptoms: "headache, fatigue, irritability, lassitude, insomnia, burning of the eyes, difficulty of concentration, and impaired judgment." Other less frequently reported symptoms related to high air-pollution levels include "frequent urination, perspiration, epigastric distress, constipation, diarrhea, low back pain, impotence, frigidity, and other types of sexual inadequacies."

Of course, Dr. La Verne recognized that not all of these symptoms can be attributed solely to polluted air. However, he felt that a significant relationship is demonstrable.

The Poisonous Pollutants

What, exactly, is in the witches' brew that most of us have to breathe? Primarily, the substances that pollute our air are the *sulfur oxides, nitric oxide, nitrogen dioxide, carbon monoxide, ozone,* and the tiny particles of dust, soot, and ash we call *particulate matter.*

In most large American cities, as much as 100 tons of *particulate matter* either fall to the ground or are breathed in by local inhabitants each day. This involves an astronomical number of individual particles, because their dimensions are measured in microns. (A micron is 1/25,000 of an inch.) The heavier particles tend to drop to the ground and therefore, except in spots very close to their source, do not present a breathing problem. But particles of less than one micron, usually called aerosols, remain suspended in the air.

These tiny particles are the real health troublemakers. They penetrate deep into the lungs and stay there, as do the particulates in tobacco smoke. A New York pathologist remarks, "On the autopsy table you can tell. The person who spent his life in the Adirondacks, and didn't smoke, has pink lungs. Those of the city dwellers, both smokers and nonsmokers, are coal black."

The worst health effects of particulates are created not so much by the particles themselves as by the chemicals they bring along with them. Among the worst of the pollutants are the *sulfur oxides*, which come mainly from industrial sources that burn fuel oil and coal.

There are many localized pockets of high sulfur oxide pollution. If the number of sulfur oxides rises to 8 to 12 parts per million (ppm) your eyes will water and you'll start to cough. Studies show that if a population is exposed to 1.5 parts per hundred million over a one-year period, an increase in cardiac and respiratory diseases occurs. Some studies show that deaths of elderly patients increase and that pulmonary disease rates climb significantly when sulfur dioxide levels reach 0.25 ppm. A research program that followed eighty-four asthmatic cases on a daily basis for one year found a 300-percent increase in acute asthmatic episodes on high-sulfur days.

Nitric oxide is largely a product of automobile engines and high-heat processes that go on in power plants and certain industrial establishments. Nitric oxide alone is not very harmful, but once it gets into the air, varying amounts of it become *nitrogen dioxide* (NO_2), which is very dangerous indeed. It is the only visible pollutant: it's yellow-brown in color and creates the smog that marks high-pollution days in urban areas. It has an odor variously described as "sweetish" or "stinging" that becomes noticeable at 1 to 3 ppm—a not unusual level.

There's a lot of this noxious substance in the air over urban areas. Researchers from the National Center for Atmospheric Research in Boulder, Colorado, wandered about rural Michigan and clambered around in the Rockies bearing sensitive monitoring equipment. They found that relatively uncontaminated air contains less than 0.25 parts per billion of nitrogen oxides. In smog-alert situations as much as 8,000 times this "clean air background" amount has been measured!

The effects of this highly visible pollutant are numerous. At concentrations of 5 to 10 ppm it definitely causes eye and nose irritation in some people. Prolonged exposure to 10 to 40 ppm can trigger emphysema attacks. Flare-ups of bronchitis can result from exposure to 50 to 100 ppm. Various experiments carried out in the late seventies indicate that the serious effects of this pollutant are greater than had previously been thought. Dr. Daniel Menzel, a Duke University researcher, postulates that breathing NO_2 affects the hormones that help regulate oxygen absorption and fluid balance in the lungs.

Most people are familiar with the harmful pollutant *carbon monoxide* (CO). It has a well-deserved reputation as a "silent killer." However, though greater concentrations of it than of any other gaseous air pollutant are found in urban atmosphere, there is still controversy about its effect on the human body. A molecule of carbon monoxide has 210 times the affinity for joining with red blood cells as does ordinary oxygen. Breathing it reduces the amount of oxygen reaching body cells, since the oxygen is "crowded out" by the carbon monoxide. However, it has to be inhaled in large quantities to result in the ultimate oxygen starvation that brings on death. Nine parts of CO per million is an allowable intake over an eight-hour period; 35 ppm breathed for one hour is not considered dangerous. A 20-ppm ratio is common in heavy traffic.

The effects of carbon monoxide on our health are, oddly enough, still a matter of dispute. There is a certain amount of this form of oxygen in our blood, generally 2 percent in the case of nonsmokers, as much as 5 percent in heavy smokers. Researchers believe that a certain tolerance for it is achieved, but that a constant level above 5 percent can be damaging. Tests show that in some persons amounts above 2 percent result in a measurable effect on vision. The same level seems to affect reaction time in some individuals. Investigators suspect that it produces more results than they are able to measure. "Threshold value below which there is no effect may not even exist," says

N. Balfour Slonin, director of the Cardiopulmonary Diagnostic Laboratory in Denver.

For people with chronic ailments, CO presents a definite menace, particularly to those suffering from heart disease. Physicians pinpoint it as the agent in 690,000 cases of angina chest pains in Los Angeles in a single year. In many cities it has been observed that fatal heart attacks are "significantly more frequent" when levels of CO go higher than 10 ppm for a period of twelve hours or more.

The most dangerous pollutant of all is the form of oxygen known as *ozone*—O_3. An ordinary oxygen molecule has two atoms; ozone has three. It's this extra atom that makes ozone such a troublemaker. It is considered so virulent that it is commonly used as the key factor in triggering a pollution alert. The presence of 0.5 ppm is enough to call for an alert, 1 ppm brings about the second alert, and when the count reaches 1.5 ppm the situation is rated serious enough to warrant the closing of factories and the halting of traffic. Fortunately, this is more of a theoretical condition than one that actually occurs. About the highest the ozone rating has gone in American cities, however badly polluted, is 1 ppm.

What does ozone do that's so bad? Inhaling it in amounts as low as 0.5 ppm can create a variety of nasty symptoms, including coughing, headache, choking, and a "dead tired" feeling. It affects breathing. Tests show that even one hour of exposure to 0.5 ppm can cause breathing difficulties, and that above 0.5 ppm visual acuity decreases and muscular coordination diminishes. No wonder the maximum concentration acceptable over an eight-hour period is considered to be 0.1 ppm.

Checking Up on Air Pollution

Fortunately, states and cities are trying to do something about air pollution, and in many areas things are better than they used to be.

In 1975, the President's Council for Environmental Quality began to look into the wild confusion that existed then in reporting air-pollution conditions. The council termed what it found "a serious national communications problem." It discovered that no less than fourteen different methods were used by local, state, and national agencies to calculate air-pollution indexes, with forty-four different words used to describe air quality.

To bring some order out of the chaos, the Federal Interagency Task Force on Air Quality Indicators was organized. It brought together the Council on Environmental Quality (CEQ), the Environmental Protection Agency (EPA), the National Oceanic and Atmospheric Administration (NOAA), the Bureau of Standards, and the Office of Environmental Affairs. They came up with the "Pollutants Standards Index" (PSI). It takes the five most prevalent and dangerous pollutants and gives "index values" to various concentrations of them.

However, the Task Force still needs to find a way to make the PSI understandable to the average citizen.

In some cities now, and supposedly in an ever-increasing number of cities in the future, our TV weathercasts and our newspapers will report the *average* index value (see chart on pages 106–7) for a particular day.

There is a difficulty with using averages. Suppose the carbon monoxide level was way up there at 500—the "significant harm" point. This is the level at which the ill and the elderly can become so sick they will actually die, and even healthy people will experience severe symptoms that can affect their normal activity. And yet, if the other four pollutants measured are all very low—for instance, at a 100 level (the level that meets the National Ambient Air Quality Standard)—the average of one 500 reading and the four 100 readings together will be a reading just above the 200 level. So what happens? Your community calls that an "alert," not the "disaster" it should be labeled.

There is considerable difference in how people are supposed to conduct themselves at these two levels of pollution. An alert warns the elderly and persons with heart or lung disease to stay indoors and reduce physical activity. But at the "disaster" level (the term is ours, not that of the Task Force; they call it the "significant harm" point) "*all* persons should remain indoors, keeping windows and doors closed. *All* persons should minimize physical exertion and avoid traffic."

If your community does have a day like the one we described (with the carbon monoxide level at 500, the rest at 100), you can hope it will have sense enough to forget about the other four pollutants and not do any averaging. If it gave all the weight to the carbon monoxide on that day, the index would rise to its highest value—and you would at least be properly warned about the danger.

You can fight for more and better-located monitoring stations in your community. If your newspaper doesn't tell you where the air-pollution monitoring stations in your city are located, a call to City Hall should bring forth that information. (Newspapers *should* print this information daily, in either list or map form.) You can also find out if mobile units are used to make spot checks on air quality at other points in the city.

In Albuquerque we found that one of the monitoring stations was "out at the City Yards," which are north of the city limits. Needless to say, if the monitoring stations are not located where the bulk of the people are, the readings are not too meaningful. The placement of such stations can result in some misleading and generalized information being given out. For example, in one western city that had several fixed monitoring stations, it took a mobile survey to alert the community to the fact that a part of the city formerly considered a highly desirable place to live actually had—because of its relationship to shopping centers, freeways, prevailing winds, and so forth—air so bad so much of the time that it presented "danger" for pregnant women, small children, and the elderly.

Another problem with the PSI is that it is based on short-term health effects. This means that, while there may not be much harm done to your health in any one twenty-four-hour period from an index of 100 (which even the NAAQS terms "moder-

POLLUTANTS STANDARDS INDEX

		Pollutant Levels				
		(in micrograms per cubic meter)				(in milligrams per cubic meter)
Index Value	Air Quality Level	Total Suspended Particulates (24-hour)	Sulfur Dioxide (24-hour)	Ozone (1-hour)	Nitrous Oxide (1-hour)	Carbon Monoxide (8-hour)
500	Significant harm	1,000	2,620	1,200	3,750	57.5
400	Emergency	875	2,100	1,000	3,000	46.0
300	Warning	625	1,600	800	2,260	34.0
200	Alert	375	800	400†	1,130	17.0
100	NAAQS*	260	365	160	§	10.0
50	50% of NAAQS	75‡	80‡	80	§	5.0
0		0	0	0	0	0

* National Ambient Air Quality Standard.
† 400 micrograms per cubic meter used instead of the ozone alert level of micrograms per cubic meter.

Where to Live for Your Health

Health Effect Description	General Health Effects	Cautionary Statements
	Premature death of ill and elderly. Healthy people will experience adverse symptoms that affect their normal activity.	All persons should remain indoors, keeping windows and doors closed. All persons should minimize physical exertion and avoid traffic.
azardous	Premature onset of certain diseases in addition to significant aggravation of symptoms and decreased exercise tolerance in healthy persons.	Elderly and persons with existing diseases should stay indoors and avoid physical exertion. General population should avoid outdoor activity.
ery unhealthful	Significant aggravation of symptoms and decreased exercise tolerance in persons with heart or lung disease, with widespread symptoms in the healthy population.	Elderly and persons with existing heart or lung disease should stay indoors and reduce physical activity.
nhealthful	Mild aggravation of symptoms in susceptible persons, with irritation symptoms in the healthy population.	Persons with existing heart or respiratory ailments should reduce physical exertion and outdoor activity.
oderate		
ood		

Annual Primary NAAQS.
No index values reported at concentration levels below those specified by "Alert Level" criteria.　　　　　　　　　　　　　　(Environmental Protection Agency)

ate," you'll notice, not "good"), the effects on you of long-term exposure to such levels could well be something worse than "moderate."

Unfortunately, it's not easy for the ordinary citizen to get truly reliable information about air pollution in his own community. It is something of a shock to find just how difficult and confusing it is. You can call City Hall, or the Department of Health, or the Environmental Health Department, or whatever other agency might seem appropriate, and try to get specific information about the locations of monitoring points and just what pollutants are checked (all communities don't check on all pollutants!), but even this is insufficient. If you do obtain the information, it's only going to give you, in most situations, figures for the average pollution in a given twenty-four-hour period.

Can You Escape Bad Air?

Is there anyplace you can go to find clean, pure air to breathe? If you don't have to earn a living there are wilderness areas where the air is cleaner. If there were any United States city with really clean air, so many of us would rush there that it would, very quickly, end up just as polluted as the dirtiest cities are now. There's a joke about the last lungful of clean air in the forty-eight contiguous states having been inhaled near Flagstaff, Arizona, some years ago.

Whatever specific information you obtain can be used as a starting point from which you can do some investigating and decision making of your own. You can profit by using your common sense and following a few general rules. The first rule is to realize that localized differences do exist—from section to section of a city, from street to street, from block to block. If you have any choice, you'd be better off not to live . . .

• near a freeway. Persons living one block from a busy highway can be subjected to hundreds of times more pollution than those a few blocks farther away.

• near a shopping center, especially downwind from it, where large numbers of cars stop, start, and idle in parking lots and at drive-up windows.

• on a corner with a stoplight.

• close to, and downwind from, a power plant, even one equipped with the best antipollution devices. It may require miles of separation to give you the protection you would have on the upwind side at a much closer spot.

• near anyplace where fixed instrument readings show high levels of any pollutant—even if they show them for only one kind of pollutant at certain times of the day.

Neither should you patronize parks, playgrounds, or playing fields that are close to or downwind from sources of pollution. If you're a jogger or a bicyclist be careful where you carry out either of these activities. Running or cycling along with automobile traffic can seriously damage your health. Adults and children at play, or exercising in other ways, breathe more deeply and thus take in more pollutants than persons who are not exerting themselves.

If you are thinking of moving to some other city or area and would like to make a sort of general check on air quality there, you can contact the Department of Health of the state or of the city. The department will either provide you with the information you'd like or tell you which other state or local agency can.

Taking refuge indoors is no solution to the problem. One might assume it is, since, when pollution levels get high enough, we are advised to "stay indoors and shut all doors and windows." However, EPA studies show that in both urban and suburban houses and apartments pollution levels are frequently "as high as that of outside air." Some contaminants are bound to sneak in from outside. You are also endangered by pollution that originates *inside* your home. In a study of dwellings in different sections of the country, researchers found that "air pollution indoors is frequently worse than pollution outdoors, and possibly more hazardous to health because most people spend far more time indoors."

Ordinary house dust is often a mix of harmful chemicals,

containing, among other substances, lead, vinyl chloride, asbestos fibers, and particulates. Sources of pollution originating inside the home include gas appliances, fireplaces and wood-burning stoves, aerosols, and cigarette smoke. Of course, by checking appliances, fireplaces, and stoves, and their vents, pipes, and chimneys, and by banning aerosols and smoking, you can eliminate a lot of pollution. Electronic air cleaners can be used to get rid of more.

That Other Pollutant—Radioactivity

A lot of us are becoming increasingly concerned about what the American Lung Association calls "the newest contaminant of all"—radioactive pollution resulting from the use of nuclear fuels. Those Americans who live near nuclear reactors are the most worried. Their fear is that our scientists and technologists don't even know what it might do. Are the fears justified?

The environmentalists and other scientists who worry about the dangers of nuclear power plants aren't nearly so concerned about the possibility of some great "China syndrome" disaster as they are about the small amounts of radiation that leak into the air on a day-to-day basis. There is a lot of argument about just how great these emanations are. Do they reach a dangerous level around the power plant, not from any accident, but simply as a result of the plant's ordinary operation?

The Nuclear Regulatory Commission, the federal organization charged with nuclear safety, says that they must be kept "as low as practicable." Which means, say many concerned scientists, that the NRC is admitting that there *are* radiations and that it is *not* judging them by health standards.

However, the basic controversy is whether the health standards themselves are adequate. Low levels of radiation once thought to be harmless are now being revealed as having unexpected dangers, some arising from the very fact that they *are* so low! These low-level "safe" dosages may be causing not only cancer but other diseases as well.

Dr. Alice Stewart, an epidemiologist who, with Dr. George Kneale, a biostatistician, conducted a long-term study of 35,000 people who worked or had worked at the Hanford, Washington, nuclear power plant, points out that "radiation is a nonspecific poison that tears tissues apart. It has, by definition, cancer and noncancer effects." She uses the "broken plate" analogy to vividly —and shockingly—explain what happens. A slightly damaged cell, she says, is like a broken plate. Though it can be glued back together again, "its integrity will never be as good as that of the original. Every time it is stressed, it will be more likely than the original to break." In the same way, a repaired cell will be "more prone to assault from both disease and physical injury than the original."

Knowing that this repair process does occur in the human body, scientists may have been lulled into a false sense of security about the possible effects of low-level radiation. If a slightly damaged cell repaired itself, even though slowly, why worry?

There's plenty of reason to worry, Dr. Stewart asserts. "When a damaged cell reproduces it can pass on the damage by sexual reproduction, or 'copy' the damaged cell and incubate these copies or clones, thereby weakening the body. Exposure to low dosages can lead to more damage than single larger doses received all at once." In the massive dose received at once, the cell is totally destroyed, and thus does not reproduce itself, creating weakened cells in the body.

One reason for the lack of concern about low-level radiation has been the view that, since mankind has always lived without ill effect with a certain amount of background radiation in his natural environment, there's no reason to fear a little additional low-level radiation.

Many scientists disagree with this opinion. Among them is Dr. Edward A. Martell, an environmental radiochemist with the National Center for Atmospheric Research in Boulder, Colorado. He points out that the natural alpha-radiation emitters, such as polonium 210, which you get all the time in water, food, and in dust in the air you breathe, are promptly dissolved in the lungs. There are billions of cells in the tissues of the lungs, and they are each, as Dr. Martell explains it, exposed to this low uniform dosage of natural alpha radiation every day. Fortunately, the emitters do not stay in the lungs. After they dissolve they are distributed in fluids that carry them throughout the body. The risk of cancer resulting from this flow of alpha radioactivity through our bodies is slight.

But there's a problem. Some of these natural alpha-radiation emitters are converted from particles that do dissolve into particles that do *not* dissolve. This happens in certain industrial processes (which is why we try to control the emissions from factory smokestacks) and as a result of forest fires. It also happens in the human lung to people who smoke.

Sometimes these insoluble alpha particles stay lodged in lung tissues for up to two years. And they can remain for decades in the lymph nodes, liver, and bones, irradiating cells with their deadly emanations.

It is estimated that a single gram of tissue containing a cluster of these insoluble particles is exposed to as much as 10,000 times the amount of radiation that would be received from natural soluble particles. It is a terrible fallacy, Dr. Martell and many other scientists believe, not to recognize the difference between the two kinds of particles. Acceptance of standards based on the assumption that their effect is the same is exposing millions to dangerous radiation.

Other scientists point out that there is still another hidden hazard in what seemed a "safe" level of radiation. The problem is that a given amount of radiation does not affect everybody to the same degree. A study by Dr. Irwin Bross, of Roswell Park Memorial Institute, brings out a disturbing new thought in the "three switches" theory. This researcher points out that the final onset of a malignancy or other disease may require a series of events, similar to the throwing of three electrical switches connected in series. These switches may be tripped by viruses, bacteria, chemicals, mechanical damage, or radiation.

An example of the disastrous way this multiple-switch effect could work out can be shown by the hypothetical case of a child who has been exposed to diagnostic X rays before birth. This gives him a 40- to 50-percent greater risk of dying from leukemia. One switch thrown. Now suppose the same child develops an allergic disease, such as asthma, before the age of four. Two switches thrown. If the child had not had the *in utero* X-ray exposure his risk of falling victim to leukemia would have been 300 to 400 percent greater than that of children who had not been exposed to the X rays. However, this particular child, with two switches thrown, now stands a *5,000-percent* increase in risk of dying from leukemia!

For such an individual, the throwing of the third switch—such as exposure to additional radiation, or even certain eating or smoking habits—could be the detonating agent that brings about his death.

It is advisable to avoid living near a nuclear reactor, or even in any highly industrial area, if you are a smoker; you're of childbearing age and expect to have children; you have young children; you or members of your family are elderly; you or members of your family have a history of illness involving frequent exposure to medical X rays; you have any chronic respiratory disease.

Lastly, if the place you live makes you fearful or worried, if it causes you to live in a state of anxiety even though neither you nor any member of your family falls into any of the above categories, you should certainly think about moving, for living with fear can be a great hazard to your health.

11

Is Your Water Safe to Drink?

Despite the continual polluting of our rivers, streams, lakes, and even our oceans, most of us assume that the water we drink almost anywhere in the country is pure and safe (unlike the water you may get when traveling abroad!). Unfortunately, this is not the case. You should worry about the water you are drinking.

The problem is not organisms. American water systems have long had those under reasonable control; chlorine does kill them. Although, as various outbreaks of gastroenteritis indicate, bacterial contamination does still occur, the pressing concern is with chemicals from industrial sources that get into the water, some of them poured into our rivers, others carried through the air by prevailing winds, often for long distances, and then deposited, sometimes in "acid rain"—rain that carries a high sulfuric and nitric acid content.

Some of the reasons for concern about the water we drink are indicated by recent revelations:

• In 1969 the U.S. Public Health Service surveyed 1,000 community water systems and discovered that 85 percent of them had *no procedure whatsoever for testing the water supply.* The

114   *Where to Live for Your Health*

Environmental Defense Fund (EDF) reports, more than a decade later, that the situation is little changed.

• A national survey shows 50,000 chemical dumps in the United States. Many of them, particularly in eastern states, are leaking poisons into underground water supplies.

• An EPA official says that hundreds of western water supply systems may be excessively radioactive because of contamination by uranium.

• In the drinking water of eighty major American cities, the EPA has found 253 (!) kinds of organic chemicals. The effects of most of them are unknown and many are believed to be harmless, but some are definitely suspected of being injurious to human health.

The Chemical Culprits

It was not until 1974 that Congress belatedly passed the Safe Drinking Water Act, a bill that, although long backed by environmentalists, had been stalled before then. The act required standards to be set for water systems serving more than twenty-five people. When it went into effect in 1977, it used a National Academy of Sciences study to help establish limits on the amounts of 16 chemicals (of the 253) which the EPA stated "pose a significant health risk of human cancer and other chronic effects."

Following is a list of these chemicals, and a discussion of some of the problems associated with them, along with the Maximum Contaminant Levels (MCLs) set for each.

Arsenic (0.05 per liter). You get more arsenic in the food you eat every day than you do from the water you drink. One source is the pesticides and herbicides that are sprayed on vegetables and fruit and that also become lodged in most animal meat. In quantity, arsenic is a deadly poison. However, some nutritionists argue that it is also a necessary nutrient. Many medical authorities are convinced that the MCL is set much too high, maintaining that it fails to allow for all the other possible sources.

Some arsenic compounds are absorbed by the gastrointestinal tract, the lungs, and the skin and become distributed throughout the body's tissues and fluids. Arsenic can accumulate in bones, muscle, skin, and human hair. In addition to latent effects, arsenic poisoning symptoms include fatigue, loss of energy, impairment of gastrointestinal function, neurological disturbances, kidney and liver dysfunctions, and skin problems.

Barium (1 mg per liter). Barium is not a problem chemical in most drinking water. It is rarely found in amounts above the MCL. You get this substance, which is not required by the body, in drinking water and from the air, but not in food. It is potentially dangerous because it may affect the gastrointestinal tract, the central nervous system, the blood vessels, and the muscles, including the heart. However, it is usually readily excreted and it is not believed that it accumulates in the body.

Cadmium (0.01 mg per liter). Cadmium comes mostly from food and tobacco, but it is also present in some drinking water. It gets there from geological sources, corrosion of iron water pipes that are zinc-galvanized, and industrial wastes, particularly from smelters. Its presence in water in any large quantity is a matter of concern to health authorities. Both zinc and calcium, which are essential elements, may protect against cadmium toxicity. Cadmium poisoning causes intense pain because of loss of bone minerals and consequent softening of the bones. Studies in humans as well as animals indicate that after ingestion cadmium also is absorbed into body tissues and then stored mostly in the kidneys and liver and is excreted at an extremely slow rate.

Chromium (0.05 per liter). This is an essential trace element you need in your diet. It is present in the air, in soil, and in some food, especially food cooked in stainless steel pans, from which it picks up some of the substance. Tests show that industrial workers who come in contact with chromium develop irritation of mucous membranes and a variety of respiratory, gastrointestinal, lung, and skin complications. The level set for allowable amounts in drinking water is only 1/1000 of the no-observed-adverse-health-effect amount, but chromium, in the opinion of many medical researchers, must be viewed with suspicion until its carcinogenic potential is more fully known.

Lead (0.05 mg per liter). Lead is a substance that particularly alarms medical authorities. There's a lot of it in our environment —in the air, put there by gasoline additives and emanations from lead storage batteries, and in the food we eat. One of the problems connected with it is that intake amounts vary greatly among individuals. There is vastly more lead in urban areas than in rural ones. The amount of it in water is affected by the acidity, hardness, and organic content of the water. Water as it comes out of the tap may have much more lead in it than water at the purification plant, for if water is slightly acidic it can dissolve lead in household piping and soldered joints.

Lead tends to accumulate in human and animal tissues. Its major toxic effects include anemia, neurological dysfunction, and liver and kidney impairment. It apparently interferes with certain enzyme activities, including ones that help in the production of red blood cells. Is it carcinogenic? Tests on humans seem to indicate that it isn't, but high concentrations do cause liver cancer in rats. Many experts think the MCL is set much too high in view of the much larger amounts of it some individuals are ingesting from water and other sources.

Mercury (0.002 per liter). One of the most toxic of all the chemical contaminants, mercury can get into drinking water from industrial sources. Large amounts of it can cause irreversible damage to the nervous system, the gastrointestinal tract, the kidneys, and the liver. Fortunately, it is a rare contaminant in drinking water in the United States, and standards for the allowable amounts are set so low that it need not be a subject of worry.

Nitrate (10.0 mg per liter). Nitrogen is found in many places in nature. It's the major component of the air we breathe and is present in soil, in plants, and in animals. In water, nitrogen tends to become the chemical nitrate. Most of it that gets into the human system is excreted, some of it in saliva. High intakes of nitrate are hazardous under conditions that are favorable to the conversion of nitrate to nitrite. Nitrite in the bloodstream causes impairment of oxygen transport. Serious poisonings in infants have occurred following the drinking of water having concentrations of more than 10 mg of nitrate-nitrogen per liter. Note that the MCL for nitrogen is set at exactly this level—10 mg— which is ten times greater than the 1 mg that is considered safe for infants. Researchers think the MCL is perfectly safe for adults, but are raising questions about the amount of nitrates that a person may get in food. There is a possibility that substances present in food may react with nitrate to create carcinogenic substances.

Selenium (0.01 mg per liter). This is one of the trickiest of the substances covered by MCL regulations. It's a trace element that you get in food but is extremely toxic if ingested in quantities of 0.1 to 10 mg per kilogram of food. Selenium poisoning can damage the gastrointestinal tract, the central nervous system, teeth, skin, lungs, kidneys, and liver. It is present in some amount in all water, but the concentration varies greatly. In some places it has been found to be 100 times the MCL, having reached the water supply from industrial wastes. "More research is necessary," is the judgment of many public health authorities.

Silver (0.05 mg per liter). Silver has no place in the human diet and is not a problem in drinking water because it is present in such insignificant amounts. In experiments with rats, large amounts ingested have resulted in liver, kidney, and spleen damage. However, the amount administered was far above the MCL set for drinking water.

Fluoride (1.4 to 2.4 mg per liter). Fluoride is the only substance with an MCL range that is variable. That is because its presence in water must be based on temperature; the activity of fluoride in the body is much greater in warm weather. There isn't much quarrel with the MCL for fluoride because medical people are not particularly worried about the health effects of any quantity you are likely to get in your drinking water, even at levels that vastly exceed the MCL. Very large doses of fluoride can cause a mottling of the enamel of the teeth and, rather more bizarre, a similar mottling of the skeletal bones. And while it may bother you to think of your bones turning brown, all experts insist there are no other effects beyond the discoloration. Unless, that is, you were to ingest 20 mg per day for twenty years or more. In that case, they say, you might suffer some crippling consequences.

Fluoride is, of course, deliberately added to the drinking water of many cities to prevent dental decay, a procedure that has been in effect for more than thirty years. A study in two Texas cities, one with a high natural level of fluoride (much above the present MCLs) and the other with an unusually low natural level, revealed no differences whatsoever in the death rate incidence of any diseases between the two cities. The American Academy of Pediatricians, the American Cancer Society, the American Dental Association, and the American Medical Association are among the organizations that support drinking-water fluoridation programs as being a safe and effective way to distribute the enamel-strengthening fluorides.

Herbicides. Only two of this class of organic compounds have been assigned MCLs—2,4-D (0.1 mg per liter) and 2,4,5-TP (0.01 mg per liter). Various studies have shown that these two defoliants, if ingested during pregnancy, tend to "produce physically or functionally defective offspring." They are not believed to be carcinogenic. The MCL for them is based on the concept that 20 percent of the daily intake of these substances will be from drinking water, the other 80 percent coming from food.

Insecticides. Only four of these organic compounds have been assigned MCLs. That doesn't mean that those not rated are necessarily harmless. It means either that their general use has already been banned, or that "not enough is known about their presence in drinking water."

Of the four with MCLs, lindane (0.004 mg per liter) is a known animal carcinogen, and endrin (0.0002 mg per liter) is suspected. Methoxychlor (0.1 mg per liter) and toxaphene (0.005 mg per liter) are evidently not carcinogens. The reason these substances are to be feared, whether cancer-causing or not, is that they accumulate in body fat after being absorbed through the lungs, the gastrointestinal tract, or the skin. Muscle spasms, dizziness, and convulsions are some of the known symptoms of poisoning by these organics.

How Safe Is "Safe Water"?

Do the MCLs allow too much of these regulated contaminants to stay in drinking water that is labeled "safe"? Many medical researchers believe that right down the line the MCLs should be reduced—in some cases drastically. They base this contention on several doubts about the standards.

One major charge is that the MCLs are not necessarily based on health considerations at all. The limits for chromium are a case in point. Before the MCLs were established, reports indicated that many municipal wells had a chromium level of around 0.05 mg per liter. Those wells would have been put out of business if the limit were set at, say, 0.04 mg per liter. So where was the limit set? At 0.05. Whether this factor of expediency was widely applied in setting the MCLs for this and other contaminants cannot be proved, and certainly it cannot be asserted that health factors were ignored. The scientists who established the MCLs argue that there were no data indicating that they should be set lower, even though some environmentalists suggest that the MCLs may have been selected with an eye to the "disproportionately high cost" of reducing a given contaminant to a lower level.

Suppose, says Dr. Frances S. Sterrett, professor of chemistry at Hofstra University, that a contaminant level is set at a point that will cause only 0.01 percent of those exposed to it to suffer some ill effects. The agency supplying the water saves some money at an apparently small health cost. How small? Well, only 20 people in a community of 200,000 might suffer some health problem. In a metropolitan area with 7 million people, 700 of them would be affected. As Dr. Sterrett points out, "For *those* people there is a 100-percent risk!"

Dr. Sterrett also suggests that as the measurement techniques for the detection of contaminants in drinking water become more sensitive, the number of compounds found will increase. "It is of paramount importance," she insists, "to develop primary drinking-water regulations, even on an interim basis, for many toxic organic chemicals as soon as possible."

Another problem in setting standards for drinking water is that all people do not drink the same amount of water. In setting the standards it was assumed that average water intake is 2 liters per day. What about the person who habitually drinks more? It has been observed that adult water consumption ranges from as little as 1.5 liters to as much as 8 liters, depending on such factors as body weight, occupation, and climate. ("Water" includes tea, coffee, soft drinks, and so forth.) Actual average consumption, according to the National Academy of Sciences study, is 1.6 liters, and it is argued that the 2-liter allowance provides enough margin of safety. The Environmental Defense Fund doesn't think it does and recommends that a change in MCLs should be made on this basis alone, if not for other reasons.

One of those "other reasons" is that the MCLs have been established for only sixteen chemicals. Might there not be other dangerous contaminants in our water? "Oh, definitely," asserted a biologist-chemist-water expert in charge of the water-testing labs of one western city. "There are several other things, particularly organics, that we should be checking for, but aren't—PCBs, for instance."

According to recent EPA disclosures, hundreds of water-supply systems in perhaps as many as fifteen western states have been tainted by uranium—both because of its natural presence and through the mining operations that get it out of the ground. The 7,500 residents of the Fairmount area, near Denver, have learned that for years they have been drinking water with high radiation levels because of the presence of a nearby uranium mine. The annual radiation dose to their bone cells is 3,000 mg, about *sixty times* the amount the average American receives from small amounts of naturally occurring radioactivity in water and food. An EPA regional director in Denver says, "I wouldn't drink it. I would go to bottled water." Yet the Safe Drinking Water Act does nothing to govern radiation levels.

Still another complaint directed against the MCLs—possibly the most damaging one of all—is that their medical basis is unsound. They're largely based on animal studies. Is the danger of contaminants to animals greater or less than it is to humans? The life expectancy of humans, for example, is thirty-five times that of mice, and people have much more varied and complex genetic backgrounds. Is the effect of exposure spread over many years for humans in any way similar to the effect of a short-term massive dose on mice?

It is the contention of medical environmentalists that the MCLs should be made much more stringent. They point out that we are all exposed to a wide variety of chemical carcinogens —in the air, in food additives, in drugs. Cancer specialists estimate that 80 to 90 percent of human cancer is caused by environmental agents, most of which are synthetic chemicals. What about their cumulative effect? Is the extra amount of them you might get in your drinking water the proverbial straw that might break the camel's back, might trigger cancer?

Can Drinking Water Be Improved?

Underlying all the challenges to the adequacy of the MCLs— and to standards for other chemicals for which limits have not yet been established—is the question: Does the technology exist to get the contaminants down to levels even the most concerned environmentalists will consider acceptable? To answer that question you must look at the various methods for cleaning up drinking water.

The basic method in use today calls for filtering water through a sand bed and then treating the filtered water with chloride to kill the bacteria that have not been filtered out. Since 1908, when it was first applied in Jersey City, New Jersey, this has been the procedure. In general it has worked pretty well against what has always been considered the main contaminant in water—bacterial agents that cause such diseases as cholera, typhoid, and dysentery. Citizens might complain about the taste of heavily chlorinated water, but at least health authorities were able to assure them that the water was safe to drink.

However, this combination of sand filter and chlorine doesn't eliminate possibly dangerous chemicals, and the chlorine itself presents chemical dangers. It produces chloroform—a substance found in the water of all eighty cities checked by the EPA—when organic substances in the water react with chlorine.

Methods do exist for overcoming these problems, but they are expensive and not widely employed. One is to use, instead of chlorine, a related compound, chlorine dioxide, which does not combine with organic chemicals. Another method involves the use of ozone. An electric current is passed through the water, resulting in a change of the molecular structure of the oxygen in the water and the creation of ozone gas. When bubbled through the water supply it both disinfects against bacteria and decreases various chemicals. Widely used in Europe and by soft-drink bottlers in this country, it is being adopted by some cities in the United States.

A third method is considered by many to be the most promising. It involves filtering not only through sand but through a bed of charcoal. However, the water must still be treated with a certain amount of chlorine.

Many authorities believe the only sure way to reduce the dangerous substances in our drinking water is to clear up the sources of contamination. That will be no small task in view of the chemical dumps and industrial establishments that are pouring their poisons into our soils, lakes, and rivers.

What Can You Do about It?

What can you do about drinking water—either in the community where you live now or in one to which you're thinking of moving?

Up to quite recently we'd have had to answer, "Not much." But, thanks to the efforts of such organizations as the Environmental Defense Fund, the League of Women Voters, and the Environmental Protection Agency, some lines of action are open. If your home community has water problems, pressure can be put on local officials to correct them. If you're moving into a new community, or thinking about doing so, you can, by your very interest in the quality of the water supply, exert pressure to get it improved.

First off, how does the water taste? If it's bad, find out why. Is the bad taste due to natural contaminants—sulfur, for example, a probably harmless substance that permeates the water in some parts of the country? Does it simply reek of chlorine used to kill a heavy infusion of bacteria that get into it from polluted sources—such as a river into which upstream communities dump their inadequately treated sewage? Or might the taste be caused by possibly dangerous chemicals that are getting into it from dumps or industrial sources?

Not all bad water is distasteful or odorous, so you can't rely solely on the taste test. Start by asking questions. Try the local office of the Environmental Protection Agency. Or call a state or local public health agency. Terminology may differ for these agencies, so if you're puzzled try City Hall—the municipal government—and ask what office you should call to find out about the water quality.

In larger cities you'll probably have no problem getting reasonably satisfying answers. Some 500 systems provide the drinking water for 65 percent of the people in the United States. You'll probably have more trouble if the community you're investigating is one of those served by the 39,500 systems that provide water for about 15 percent of the population. And the variations in these smaller systems, in the words of an EPA investigator, are "disturbing, ranging from 'hopelessly polluted' to 'beautifully clear, far better than anything you'll get in most large systems.'"

One yardstick you can use is the MCLs. Although they have their faults, as we have duly noted, they do provide a basic guide to chemical pollutants. How close does the water system you're checking out come to meeting these standards? You should hope to find that the chemical pollution is *less* than the Maximum Contaminant Levels shown in this table.

Inorganic Chemicals	*Milligrams per liter*
Arsenic	0.05
Barium	1.0
Cadmium	0.01
Chromium	0.05
Lead	0.05
Mercury	0.002
Nitrate	10.0
Selenium	0.01
Silver	0.05
Fluoride	1.4 to 2.4

Organic Chemicals	
Chlorinated Hydrocarbons (Insecticides)	
Endrin	0.0002
Lindane	0.004
Methoxychlor	0.1
Toxaphene	0.005
Chlorophenoxys (Herbicides)	
2,4-D	0.1
2,4,5-TP (Silvex)	0.01

You'll just have to take somebody's word for it that the contaminant levels are what they say they are. EPA officials admit that "we just don't have the manpower to check out more than a small percentage of the nation's water systems." One of them told us a classic tale—possibly apocryphal—of a small-town water system that was delivering chemically polluted water from a reservoir. A local official who, along with other functions, carried out the management of the water system assured the citizenry that he had cleared it all up with "carbon filtration." He accomplished this feat by rowing across the reservoir dragging a bag of charcoal.

You'll find a detailed set of guidelines for sizing up a local public water supply in a booklet provided by the EPA—*Manual for Evaluating Public Drinking Water Supplies*. You can get a free copy by sending to Water Supply Division, Environmental Protection Agency, Washington, D.C. 20460.

If you're looking into the water situation in a suburb or a rural area and find the water is supplied by one of the 30 million or so wells that provide water for 20 percent of Americans, you'll find yourself in a no-man's-land full of booby traps. Most wells have never been tested at all, and many are subject to sources of contamination that their owners never dreamed of. Septic tanks, polluted rivers, chemical dumps, and overflowing storm sewers can all contribute to pollution of wells.

The residents of Medford, a community on Long Island, discovered that the nice clean-looking water from the individual wells which supply most of the homes was loaded with carcinogenic chemicals that were seeping into the wells from nearby chemical dumps. Citizens in the community had never bothered to check their wells until, at a civic meeting, someone happened to mention that his water had been "tasting funny lately." It turned out that others present had the same complaint. Of 165 wells tested, *all* were found to be contaminated. State authorities express the fear that thousands of other private wells in the area may be equally unsafe.

If you own a property with its own well, or are thinking of buying one, or get your water from a small independent water system that hasn't been checked or about which you have some doubts or suspicions, by all means *have the water tested*. Call the county agent, or the local or county government, and ask if there's a public agency that will test a water sample you send in. If there isn't, ask for the name of a private laboratory that will do so.

Millions of people, despairing of the public water supply or the water from their own wells, have turned to buying bottled water for drinking purposes. Many others have installed devices designed to purify water. It is estimated that upwards of 2 million are sold each year. Some fit on sink counters, some under the sink, and some simply attach to the faucet. Some filter all the water; others bypass water not used for drinking. The cost ranges from under twenty-five dollars to several hundred dollars. They use different methods, including carbon filtration; distillation, which boils the water and collects the vapor; and ion exchange, in which a chemical removes calcium and other minerals.

Do they really make the water safe to drink? Are the claims by their makers backed up by performance? The answer, we're sorry to say, is "no." In some cases they don't do any good at all; in others, they actually create dangers.

Researchers at Baylor College of Medicine tested four sink-top charcoal filters. They found that in water that went through the filters and was then allowed to stand overnight, the bacteria actually *multiplied*, jumping from several hundred to 7 million per 100 ml of water. Never mind the fact that many of the bacteria counted were harmless, said the researchers in their report. Their sheer numbers indicated the ineffectiveness of the filtering system. No scientist we talked to had anything good to say about the ability of any home filtering system to remove bacteria.

How about the carcinogenic chemicals? Can any filtering system remove them? Again the answer is negative. Activated carbon can remove them from public water systems. However, in home systems the time element is left out. It takes from seven to eighteen minutes for a large-scale public system to trap most carcinogenic agents as they pass through a carbon bed three to four feet thick. Obviously, home systems have nothing like that amount of carbon, nor do they allow anything like that amount of time. The carbon bed in home systems is only one or two *inches* thick, and the water, when you turn on the tap, passes through it in a few seconds.

The systems that distill water present another hazard. They

produce clear, odorless water that is free of bacteria but not necessarily of chemical contaminants. However, their main drawback is the fact that drinking distilled water is not good for your health because it does not contain the necessary minerals that enable your body to use water correctly. The same is true of water that has been artificially softened. Water used for drinking and cooking should not go through water-softening systems.

Hard Water—Is It More Healthful?

Are there any *natural* qualities of water that make some water more healthful? For instance, is "hard" water (that is, water with more minerals in it) better for you to drink than "soft" water? It's difficult, if not impossible, to give a flat answer. Medical authorities disagree but the National Academy of Sciences reports that hard water just may reduce the risk of heart disease, high blood pressure, and stroke. Is it that the soft water is doing harm or that the hard water is doing good?

The controversy goes back to the sixties, when Dr. Henry A. Schroeder, an associate professor of clinical physiology at Dartmouth Medical School, made a study comparing the death rates in soft-water areas with those in areas having hard water. He found that there were many more deaths from cardiovascular disease in soft-water regions, such as those along the Atlantic and Pacific coasts. Hard-water areas along the Mississippi, Missouri, and Ohio rivers had lower death rates. The rate of heart-disease death in Savannah, Georgia, which has very soft water, was 826 per 100,000. In Lincoln, Nebraska, a hard-water city, heart death rate was a low 299 per 100,000.

"Some factor either present in hard water, or missing or entering in soft water, appears to affect death rates from degenerative cardiovascular disease," the Dartmouth scientist stated.

Neither he nor subsequent researchers have been able to go much further than that in their conclusions, and we would like to point to the fact that death rates in South Dakota, which has the hardest water in the nation, with 299 parts of dissolved salts to the million, are not much lower than those in Oregon, which has the softest water—17 parts per million.

Research might someday reveal the effects of hard and soft water on the arteries or the heart. Maybe, eventually, the softness or hardness of drinking water will become a medical criterion in choosing a new place to live.

12

Is Noise Making You Sick?

Acoustic engineers like to tell the story, probably apocryphal, of a woman who lived in an apartment right next to the elevated section of the New York subway in Brooklyn. A scientist studying the effects of too many decibels on the human body and psyche asked her if he could set up his sound-sensing equipment in her living room to measure the noise. Shouting above the thunder of a passing train, the accommodating lady wanted to know, "What noise?"

Many of us all too calmly accept the din that assails our ears. We may not be quite so oblivious as to ask, "What noise?" but we give scant thought to its impact on us. Most people don't even think of noise as a factor to consider when selecting a new community or neighborhood to which they might move. Whether they are moving to a distant location in the Sunbelt or just from the city to the suburbs, or vice versa, it hasn't occurred to a surprising number of people that they should stop and ask, "Wait a minute—how about the noise level?"

Yet all biometeorologists, ecologists, and medical authorities recommend that you consider noise. Living in a noisy location can make you sick, both physically and mentally. It may seriously exacerbate a chronic ailment you already have. It can be particularly hard on children and older people. Even if you're stuck where you are, it isn't as if there's nothing you can do about it.

Can You Take the Noise?

Medical researchers aren't sure that they've succeeded in cataloging all of the physical effects of noise, but they have studied enough of them to know that noise at any level creates bodily reactions.

"The idea that people get used to noise is a myth," says an Environmental Protection Agency report. "Even when we think we have become accustomed to noise, biological changes still take place inside us. . . . Noise does not have to be loud to bring on these responses. . . . It may be that our bodies are kept in a near-constant state of agitation by 'unnoticed' noise."

Among the responses referred to is an increase in blood pressure, which has been demonstrated to go up with "even moderate noise exposure." Your heartbeat definitely increases when you are subjected to any exceptionally loud noise, a reaction that can be fatal to those with impaired hearts. Another consequence of noise is an increase in the body's output of adrenaline. The most damaging medical indictment of noise is that it contributes to stress and tension.

Hospital and police records are full of cases that illustrate to what lengths people can be driven when they are bothered by noise. In Chicago an aggravated apartment dweller kept yelling at a group of boys who played in a nearby vacant lot. One day he got a gun and shot one of them. In Los Angeles a motorist jumped out of his car at a stoplight and, wielding a jack handle, smashed the windshield of the horn-honking motorist behind him. In Cleveland, an irate householder attacked a sanitation worker with a baseball bat when the noise of the garbage truck early in the morning finally got to be too much for him to take.

A psychiatrist told us that these instances of outright violence in response to noise are traceable to "irritability built up by noise exposure."

An Environmental Protection Agency report on the subject says:

Such extreme actions are not the usual responses to noise and stress. Some people cope with loud noise by directing their anger and frustration inward, by blaming themselves for being upset, and by suffering in silence. Others resort to a denial of the problem altogether, considering themselves so tough that noise does not bother them. Still others deal with noise in a more direct manner, swallowing sleeping pills and wearing ear plugs, increasing their visits to doctors, keeping their windows closed, rearranging. their sleeping quarters, spending less time outdoors, and writing letters of complaint to government officials.

Most of the time these ways of contending with noise are not likely to eliminate noise or the underlying annoyance. Short of taking extreme action—which is unlikely to solve the problem either—most people who cannot cope with noise in these ways typically direct their anger and frustration at others and become more argumentative and moody, though not necessarily violent. This noise-induced, anti-social behavior may be far more prevalent than we realize.

Noise can strain relations between individuals, cause people to be less tolerant of frustration and ambiguity, and make people less willing to help others. One recent study, for example, found that, while a lawnmower was running nearby, people were less willing to help a person with a broken arm pick up a dropped armload of books. Another study of two groups of people playing a game found that the subjects playing under noisier conditions perceived their fellow players as more disagreeable, disorganized, and threatening. Several industrial studies indicate that noise can heighten social conflicts both at work and at home. And reports from individuals suggest that noise increases tensions between workers and their supervisors, resulting in additional grievances against the employer.

Noise—Menace to Mental Health

It is difficult to get exact figures about the effects of noise on mental health. One rather striking unit of measurement is employed by UCLA researchers W. C. Meecham and H. G. Smith, who thought that mental hospital admissions would be a good indication of how a noisy airport affected the people living near it. How about comparing a neighborhood close to an airport with a relatively quiet one nearby?

The two communities they chose were in the Los Angeles area. One, Inglewood, was under the shadow of LAI, the notoriously busy—and noisy—Los Angeles International Airport. The other was El Segundo, a few miles away, where the sounds of aircraft landing and taking off are considerably less. There is little to distinguish these two communites from each other racially, economically, or socially. They're both middle-class, middle-income, ethnically balanced. The only real difference is their relationship to a major airport.

So what did the researchers find? Admissions to mental hospitals among the inhabitants of Inglewood, the airport community, run consistently *29 percent higher* than those from El Segundo, the "quiet" community! The researchers felt justified in declaring that jet racket was a decisive factor in determining the mental health of the two populations. Of course, Meecham and Smith would be the first to admit that this is only a rough criterion. There might be other factors affecting the inhabitants of the two communities studied. On the other hand, a really in-depth study of the two communities, comparing marital arguments, parent-child discord, juvenile delinquency, school truancy, and a number of other factors, might reveal that the situation in Inglewood is actually worse than the Meecham-Smith study implies. After all, most emotionally disturbed people do not reach the point where they have to be hauled off to mental hospitals.

The Meecham-Smith study is one of the very few attempts that have been made anywhere to equate severe mental disturbances with the amount of noise people are subjected to in and near their homes. It presents striking evidence that noise, in most people's minds, is a vastly underrated environmental factor in the choice of a place to live. It amazes us that people continue to buy homes near airports, busy freeways, traffic-choked shopping centers, or on super-busy street corners, paying full prices and full rentals for such properties. They ought to get big discounts to compensate them for the potential health hazards involved.

Not the least of the disastrous effects of noise is how it disturbs sleep.

"The sleeping-pill people would find their business cut in half if we could eliminate noise." The psychiatrist was being jocular when he told us that, but he was serious about the detrimental effects of noise on sleep. Many other factors contribute to the national malady of insomnia, but noise is a much bigger factor than most people realize.

Even when you are not actually awakened by noise, it can hurt you by making demands on your body to adapt. Constant or intermittent noise robs you of the kind of sleep you need. Research has shown that sounds not quite loud enough to wake you up still disturb you, causing you to shift from deep sleep to light sleep. Even though you think you have slept through the night, you may wake up still tired. You've had too small a percentage of the kind of deep sleep you need for true restoration. Elderly persons and those who are ill are more effected by this erosion of needed sleep, but persons of all ages and states of health suffer from it.

Pregnant? Beware of Noise

No one in this noisy world of ours seems to escape the baneful effects of unwanted sound—not even the unborn. "There is ample evidence that environment has a role in shaping the physique, behavior, and function of animals, including man, from conception and not merely from birth. The fetus is capable of perceiving sounds and responding to them by motor activity and cardiac rate change."

This statement by Dr. Lester Sontag, of the Fels Research Institute, indicates medical concern over the effects of noise on the unborn. An increase in heartbeat rate shows direct perception of sound by the fetus. However, the mechanism by which the unborn infant might be harmed by noise is most likely the effect it has on the mother, for when her body responds to noise, it undergoes physical changes. If noise subjects the mother to stress during the key period of fourteen to sixty days after conception, the indirect response of the fetus may threaten its development. Birth records show that in noisy areas there is a high percentage of low-weight newborn infants. Some medical researchers are convinced that there is a definite link between noise and birth defects. Studies of newborn infants born of mothers living near noisy airports reveal a disproportionate number of abnormalities such as harelip, cleft palate, and defects in the spine.

"While it cannot be said at what level maternal exposure to noise is dangerous to the fetus, these findings do create some concern," concludes one medical report. "It is known that extreme stress of any type will certainly take a toll of the fetus, but, in the case of noise, it is not known how much is required to have an effect. The risk of even a slight increase in birth defects is considerably disturbing."

Coping with Noise

What can you do about noise?

First, you must recognize that something should be done, and that the medical concern about noise is a serious one. Try to determine if noise has been bothering you more than you've wanted to admit, or more than you may have realized. Is it a potential health hazard for you or for some other member of your family who is perhaps even more affected by it than you are?

You may be able to do something at the community level. We can recommend no better first step in this direction than to take a look at Robert Alex Baron's *The Tyranny of Noise* (St. Martin's Press). It is the personal testament of a person who became an ardent anti-noise crusader with remarkable effectiveness. When jackhammer-wielding crews on a New York subway construction project made life in his apartment intolerable, Baron plunged into organizing CQC—Citizens for a Quieter City. It may not have made New York a truly *quiet* city, but it did stir the city to take some action to muffle some of the din. And it did set up a pattern for community action elsewhere. In hundreds of communities across the nation people have become more noise conscious and aware of CQC's basic contention that noise can be abated by passing—and enforcing—the right laws.

We suggest that you find out what your local or state government is doing about cutting down on noise. You can start by contacting the Department of Public Health. Even if it doesn't have a noise-abatement division (although it—or some other agency—*should* have), the people in this department will tell you the laws and regulations. Your own ears will tell you whether they're being enforced.

In taking a stand against noise, you're likely to come up against a lot of opposition. You might bear in mind Baron's advice. He suggests that to spot official justifications for noise—or indifference to it—you should be prepared to be handed the following myths: "Noise is the price of progress" . . . "Noise is a necessary evil" . . . "Noise abatement must be realistic" (that is, not cost anything) . . . "The public doesn't want to pay for quiet" . . . "Background noise is acceptable; it's the intrusive noise that is the problem" . . . "Daytime noise is more acceptable than nighttime noise."

Can You Find a Quiet Place to Live?

You should consider the allowable noise levels of any community in which you're thinking of living. These *are* quieter towns and cities; some states have passed laws that put a ceiling on noise levels. North Carolina, for example, limits daytime noise in residential areas to 60 decibels, nighttime noise to 55. Colorado puts the daytime limit at 55 decibels, the nighttime ceiling at 50. Various Colorado communities, however, have set their limits lower. The Denver suburb of Wheatridge, for instance, prohibits both daytime and nighttime noise higher than 37 decibels, one of the lowest ceilings in the nation. Coral Gables, Florida, has a 40-decibel limit on daytime noise and a low 35-decibel limit on noise at night. Boston sets its limits at 60 and 50; New York City at 65 and 45; Salt Lake City at 65 and 60. Albuquerque chose 61 and 61 for its limits, while Grand Rapids, Michigan, a city of almost the same size, has done much better, limiting its noise to 52 decibels during the day and allowing no more than 45 at night. (All of these figures are for residential areas; decibel levels allowable for commercial and industrial areas are higher.)

You'll certainly be better off if you move to a community that *tries* to make things quieter. However, that's not enough. The specific location within a community is just as important as the general allowable noise level. Live on a corner near a traffic light and no matter what the regulations, you're going to hear a lot more noise than if you lived in the middle of a block that doesn't have traffic starting and stopping at the end of it. Live anywhere near a freeway with truck traffic and you'll obviously be subjected to more diesel racket (not to mention fumes) than if you lived a few blocks away from a heavily traveled highway. Live on the leeward side of such an artery of traffic and you'll be assailed by a lot more noise than you would put up with if you lived on the windward side.

In rural locations the same rule applies: there can be great differences within short distances. We once came close to buying a recreational log cabin in a remote canyon in New Mexico. It was half a mile from the highway, across a river, and it seemed serene when we first visited it on a Sunday morning. When we came back to it later we made a horrifying discovery. Although the road was distant, traffic noises bounced off a cliff beyond it, turning the canyon into a veritable echo chamber.

We had a similar experience on a Vermont farm where we once spent a summer. The farm sprawled over 1,000 acres but, unfortunately, the house sat just a few yards from the road, no doubt to save snow plowing. This picturesque road had once been a peaceful country lane, but it had turned into a major connecting road that carried an unexpected amount of traffic. Even though we were "miles from nowhere," more cars and trucks passed our house in a day than travel on many a residential street in a large city.

Don't minimize the hazards of living near a busy airport. How near? That's the question. There are many factors to consider—the prevailing winds, the usual takeoff and landing patterns, the kinds of aircraft. Medically, sound of about 85 decibels is considered dangerous. If you're within two miles of a jetport you're in trouble, because a jet will deliver that amount of sound to the ground when it's 10,000 feet above it. You'll be subjected to annoying noise even if you're several miles away. It is estimated that the air traffic in and out of New York's John F. Kennedy Airport delivers undesirable sound levels over a 121-square-mile area. Noise from this busy international airport adversely affects millions of people!

Even country locations are subject to excessive aircraft noise, although not of the 85-decibel variety, if they happen to be located right under the normal flight path of many aircraft. And of course there are the military air bases. The noise of the big bombers and the zooming fighters is greater than that from civilian aircraft, in spite of the air force's efforts to cut the noise of its planes.

Geographic factors affect airport noise. If you move to a high-altitude city, such as Denver, Albuquerque, or Salt Lake City, you'll experience more airport noise at a given distance than you would at sea level; because of the lighter atmosphere, planes require longer takeoff runs.

Climate, too, plays a role in noise. If you live in an "outdoor climate" where you keep your windows open a substantial part of the year and spend a great deal of time in your patio or yard, of course you'll be subjected to a lot more noise from aircraft, traffic, and neighbors. Even noises that would normally be bottled up in homes—the practicing drummers and guitar players, the blaring stereos, the too-loud TVs, the clamorous kids

—will be noticeable. We've known many people who were rather surprised by this factor when they moved to the benign climate of our adopted state of New Mexico. In most areas of this state it's not necessary to shut yourself inside your quiet air-conditioned home, as it is at times in other Sunbelt locations.

There's a way to find out how much outside noise is hammering away at a home you're thinking of buying or renting—or, for that matter, at your present home. It's called the "walk-away" test. Have one person stand in a room holding some reading matter at chest level and start to read aloud in a normal voice while you back away. If you can't understand the words after you've backed up seven feet, that's bad. It means there's a lot of noise coming between you and the reader. You ought not to consider living there if you can avoid it and if you're mindful of your health.

Actually, studies indicate that you should think twice about a location where you begin not hearing the reader at a distance of twenty-five feet. The EPA rates twenty-six to seventy feet as "normally acceptable." The walk-away test is something you should try at different times of the day and night and on different days of the week to be sure you're getting the entire range of possible noise.

13

Can Climate Help Your Allergies, Asthma, Bronchitis, Sinusitis, Emphysema?

No one afflicted with an allergy that causes breathing difficulties, who suffers from frequent bouts of sinusitis, who has any chronic respiratory disease—asthma, bronchitis, or emphysema—needs to be told that factors present in the place he lives can compound his misery. If you fall into one of the above categories, you probably have considered getting away to a different climate, where what's bothering you won't be present.

Are such thoughts simply wild dreams? When you get to the promised land will the same malign influences pursue you? Or will new ones take their place to bedevil you as viciously as did the troubling factors you left behind?

What you need to do first is to find out just what it is in your present environment 'that is hurting you. Is it cold? Pollen? Humidity? Polluted air? Stormy weather? Combinations of one or more of these or other factors?

What Weather Does to Your Breathing Problems

If you have an ailment that has impaired the ability of your respiratory tract to function normally, one of your worst enemies is cold, particularly cold combined with dampness.

In one survey made among 1,500 patients with asthma and emphysema, 60 percent of them said they suffered most in "cold, rainy, foggy weather." In northern climates, the first cold spell of the year is marked by an increase in hospital admissions of persons with chronic respiratory illnesses.

Inhaling cold air has a worse effect on asthmatics than it has on people with no respiratory problem. In normal individuals the respiratory tract is astonishingly efficient at heating inhaled cold air. In one set of experiments with people having no breathing impairment it was shown that air delivered to the lips at a temperature of $-100°$ C. was heated to within one or two degrees of body temperature in the time it traveled the short distance to the trachea. Inhaling air of such a low temperature would be a disaster for an asthmatic, however. The impeded airways of asthmatics are not able to heat the air rapidly enough. When the cold air enters the bronchial tract, an asthmatic attack follows.

If you are an asthmatic your impaired respiratory system undergoes a shock every time you go from warm indoor temperatures into outdoor winter air that is twenty, thirty, or more degrees colder. Breathing passages that are already swollen clog up as the insufficiently heated air hits them. Even in bed the cold can get you. As the temperature drops during the night you get chilled—a condition responsible, doctors say, for many of the nocturnal attacks suffered by asthmatics and others with breathing problems.

Numerous medical research studies have shown that exposure to cold also increases the bodily production of histamine. So if you're allergic, the presence of histamine induced by the cold, with all the symptoms it causes, can only compound your misery.

Another weather enemy of anyone with a respiratory ailment is high humidity. Why is humidity harmful? When the humidity is high, evaporation from your body tissues is slowed down. This has the effect of speeding up your breathing rate, which in turn has the effect of reducing the carbon dioxide in the blood, because the CO_2 is blown off by the excessive breathing. When the CO_2 content of the blood is reduced, the blood becomes more alkaline. Alkalinity of the blood can bring on allergic reactions.

The negative consequences of breathing very humid air can be partly explained by the effect it has on the lungs. Your lungs play an important role in the excretion of water, ridding your body of about one-fourth as much water as do the kidneys. The lungs, of course, excrete the water as a gas or vapor, not, as do the kidneys, in liquid form. In the lungs water vapor is balanced against the water in the blood and in the air passages. Dry air helps the excretion of water vapor from swollen cells, whereas humid air impedes it, thus increasing the discomfort arising from the swollen tissues.

Another bad effect of humidity on respiratory patients is the role it plays in bronchial infections, creating a favorable environment for bacteria. Thus it aggravates many respiratory problems, particularly creating reactions in allergics sensitive to bacteria.

However, humidity is not always bad. Many individuals allergic to pollen find that they are more comfortable during periods of excessive humidity. This is not because of the humidity itself but because winds are usually calmer in humid weather and therefore they are not stirring up and distributing pollen.

Some people with respiratory problems, particularly allergics, are adversely affected by drops in atmospheric pressure. According to Dr. Harry Swartz, chief of the Allergy Clinic at New York Polyclinic Hospital, "Barometric pressure tends to keep the capillaries at normal or near normal diameter. When the pressure falls, the tendency of the allergic's capillaries is to widen. In this widening, fluid blood seeps out of the capillary walls into the surrounding tissue, thus causing a situation indistinguishable from an actual allergic reaction and symptoms."

Air Pollution and Your Respiratory Ailments

Air pollution can team up with weather factors to make life miserable for people with respiratory diseases. Worse than that, it can sometimes be lethal. Numerous studies in American cities show sharp increases in mortality among respiratory disease sufferers during times of heavy air pollution. The inversion layers that can lock pollutants into the air breathed by urban dwellers in Los Angeles, New York, Denver, and other cities are usually marked by a sharp increase in both hospital admissions and deaths.

The effect of air pollution on respiratory illness sufferers is complex, and, in the words of Dr. Manuel Lopez of Tulane University Medical School, it must "be considered as a result of the sum total of pollutants in the atmosphere in addition to other climatic factors, such as temperature, humidity, barometric pressure, and wind velocity."

The way pollutants in the air produce their bad effects is obvious. The noxious chemicals and particles act as irritants that cause sinuses and air passages to swell. They thus make breathing more difficult. When several patients in two Pennsylvania cities were examined, less breathing capacity was observed in those from the city that had the higher level of air pollution. In animal experiments it has been observed that breathing polluted air in which ozone is a major component can thicken the bronchial walls, severely limiting breathing capacity.

In an extensive study in Nashville, Tennessee, a 300-percent increase in asthma attacks was recorded during periods when there was a high sulfate level in the air. A survey in New York City revealed that at temperatures of 20° F. to 40° F. asthmatics were more affected by sulfur dioxide. At temperatures higher than this it did not seem to have a marked effect. In the New

York episode, the harm done by the polluted air was increased by the combination with cold.

Other researches have confirmed the link between cold and worsened effects of pollutants on chronic respiratory disease sufferers. A study in Utah, for example, revealed that temperatures of 30° F. or below, particularly if there was a sudden drop to that level, increased the sufferings of asthmatics.

What Climate Should You Choose?

What kind of climate should you pick if you're afflicted with a respiratory ailment? Most likely you should follow the advice of a Boston physician who told us it should be "warm instead of cold, dry instead of humid, sunny rather than cloudy, calm instead of stormy, and have clean air rather than polluted air."

Can you really find all that in one place? Well, yes—or at least almost. If, for economic reasons, you have to live in or near a city, there's no longer any place where you don't have to cope with some polluted air. In fact, some western cities have special pollution problems simply because they *are* so sunny. When we speak of smog, we usually mean the kind Los Angeles has, which results from the action of sunlight on automobile emissions. Hundreds of chemical transformations take place, creating what is known as "photochemical smog." Until we succeed in redesigning the automobile, many western cities that formerly were noted for their clean, sparkling air are going to be plagued by this kind of pollution.

But all those other desirable qualifications abound in the southwestern states. For more than a century this dry, sunny part of the country has been and continues to be a Mecca for those suffering from respiratory ills. It is widely recommended by physicians for asthma, bronchitis, emphysema, sinusitis, and hay fever patients. If you are contemplating a move because you or someone in your family suffers from any of these ailments, you certainly should—after consulting a doctor—consider this area.

However, if your respiratory problem is aggravated or caused by pollen allergies, you may not find relief in the Southwest. The very dryness, which can be beneficial for so many, can cause new torments for others. In many southwestern locations winds whip up dust from sparsely vegetated desert areas, from unpaved roads, and from construction sites—of which there are many in this fast-growing part of the country. The dust itself can be irritating, so that even if the pollen count is low, what there is will trouble you more. Doctors report that a pollen count of 50 in a dry, dusty location can have as bad an effect on some allergy sufferers as a count of 1,000 in damper climates.

While parts of the Southwest may be free of the ubiquitous nuisance of ragweed, the region has its own troublesome native plants. Sagebrush, for instance, which has such romantic western connotations, makes life miserable for many allergics. Plants growing in the Southwest, because of their harsh struggle for survival, were gifted by nature with more pollen per plant. Thus even a thinly vegetated area can cause a disproportionate amount of trouble.

Many allergics and asthmatics find the most relief in alpine climates, especially the high, green forest and meadow lands of the mountain West. The air is cleaner and drier, especially at some distance from the larger cities. But altitude alone seems to be of some help. One medical report on climate-chamber experiments at the Biometeorological Research Centre in Leiden, the Netherlands, notes that asthmatics who are "wheezy at sea level" have found that their complaints decrease or disappear altogether as soon as the 5,000-foot level is reached. The relief continues as long as the sufferer stays at high altitude, and in some cases relief lasts for several months after a return to sea level. In one study it was found that two hours in a pressure chamber with a simulated altitude of 5,000 feet brought a surprising six months of relief to some asthma victims.

There don't seem to be any statistics on how many asthmatics have found relief in high-altitude places in the West, but the number must be considerable. We personally have talked to scores.

Allergists themselves are cautious about recommending to anyone with respiratory problems that such-and-such a climate will cure his ills. There are too many combinations of factors and too many idiosyncrasies present in allergic individuals for there to be any simple answers to all the questions. For instance, while dry climates seem to help most people with breathing difficulties, humid climates are by no means ruled out. Many thousands of retirees, as well as younger people, have moved to Florida and other states in the Southeast, and to locations along the Gulf Coast—all of which are, of course, humid—and have found their breathing problems helped by the warmth. This is true even for some sinus sufferers. It seems that, for many people, humidity is most harmful when it is combined with cold. Warmer temperatures apparently minimize its effects.

That was certainly the conclusion reached by Swedish physicians who carried out an experiment that is often cited by biometeorologists. For their subjects the researchers chose ten weather-sensitive patients with chronic airway obstruction. After extensive daily tests, carried out over a period of a month, in a clinic at Gothenburg, the patients were flown to the Canary Islands. They were also tested daily in the humid, warm climate there. All of the patients reported that they felt better. And, in eight of the ten, the clinical findings showed they really *were* better, with their air passages clearer and their breathing easier. Some of the patients had suffered their attacks for more than twenty years. Their recovery, which was attributed to warmth rather than to other factors, was deemed "remarkable" by doctors and patients alike.

However, special menaces lurk for many allergy sufferers in humid air, just as for others it might be dry air that presents the problems. If you are one of the unfortunates who are allergic to molds and spores that live, grow, and multiply profusely in dampness, you will probably be miserable in a humid climate where such organisms thrive. We were recently visited by some relatives moving west from Florida, which they liked except for the dampness. None of the humans in this family had developed any particular allergy to molds, but their *dog* had. She had bare patches where her fur had been replaced by fungi of some kind and she was having expensive allergy shots. Since more kinds of molds and spores flourish in warmer climates, there's a chance you might encounter some new variety that has even more disastrous effects on you than did the ones that bothered you back home.

Before you make any kind of a move, you should be certain that what's bothering you is something in the climate—not the cat or the parakeet or house dust, or something else that a new location isn't going to help. We are often reminded of a family we knew who moved from the Midwest to Arizona for their son's asthma. The boy had suffered frequent nocturnal attacks. The family had often vacationed in the Southwest, where the boy never had any breathing difficulties. Finally they made the big move. Then came the day when the moving van arrived, bringing their furniture and other belongings. That night the boy woke up wheezing and gasping for breath. Frightened afresh, his parents rushed him to a nearby hospital. The eventual diagnosis: he was allergic to his mattress!

Never forget that for the allergic or the asthmatic, psychological factors often have serious health consequences. If you are going to take your worries with you, or if relocating is going to create new stresses for you or any member of your family, you must keep in mind that these can cause you as much trouble as the allergenic substances that trigger your attacks.

14

Can Climate Help Your Arthritis?

It is safe to say that there's probably not one among the 7 million U.S. citizens who suffer from rheumatoid arthritis—perhaps even no one among the additional millions afflicted with osteoarthritis, the kind we all get in some degree as we get older —who hasn't wondered if maybe a change of climate would help ease his or her stiffness and pain. Scientists at the National Climatic Center say they get more inquiries about arthritis, and where to go to find relief from it, than they do about any other ailment to which the human flesh is heir.

No climate will magically *cure* your arthritis, but a change of climate might *help*. Arthritis patients for whom moving from one kind of climate to another has proved beneficial often consider themselves cured, even though the disease is still present from a clinical standpoint.

What Weather Does to Your Arthritis

It has always been known that weather affects arthritics. Long before it was labeled "arthritis," people complained that "the weather has fired up my rheumatism." Medical doctors, too, were sure that there was a weather connection. But just what was it? Dampness? Wind? Cold? Storminess?

At one time or another, all of these weather phenomena have been labeled as the culprits. But the matter remained puzzling. Reactions varied from patient to patient, and even for the same patient. Sometimes there would be flare-ups clearly associated with the weather—a damp, cold spell, for example. At other times the weather might be equally damp and cold, and the patient who had complained before would seem to be unaffected.

Most puzzling of all were the cases of the "weather prophets." The sun could be shining, the sky blue, the temperature comfortable, the humidity low, yet an arthritis victim would be groaning in pain and attributing his sufferings to "a change in the weather." This phenomenon couldn't be dismissed as imagination, because it was much too common. And the arthritic who vowed he could "feel a storm coming" usually proved to be right. In twenty-four hours, more or less, the storm did arrive. Of course, scientists knew that certain meteorological changes do occur in advance of a storm (see Chapter 2, "Up and Down with the Barometer"), but doctors did not know exactly which of these changes were triggering arthritis attacks.

They no longer have to puzzle over this medical mystery. In fact, it is a mystery no longer, thanks to a classic research program carried out by Dr. Joseph Lee Hollander, an eminent rheumatologist at the University of Pennsylvania. Dr. Hollander set up a kind of laboratory in which it would be possible to study arthritis patients under controlled conditions where any possible combination of weather factors could be created.

The laboratory in the University of Pennsylvania Hospital is called the Climatron. In this fifteen-foot-square, pleasantly furnished room patients can live comfortably for long periods of time while scientists create different "climates." Controls that regulate temperature, humidity, barometric pressure, air flow, and ionization are located outside the Climatron, where they are operated without the knowledge of the occupants. The conditioned air is pumped into the room through many perforations in the ceiling and exhausted quietly through a duct near the floor. The subjects cannot hear or see any changes that are occurring in the atmosphere of the chamber.

The Patients in the Climate Chamber

The patients who took part in Dr. Hollander's pioneering experiments were all weather-sensitive arthritics who believed that weather changes worsened their symptoms. The doctors studying them carried out standard tests at intervals throughout each day. The patients' hand grips were tested for strength; the times it took for them to rise from a chair, walk across the chamber, and reseat themselves were clocked; and their joints were checked for tenderness, swelling, pain, and motion.

Supplementing the doctors' examinations were the records kept by the patients themselves. Four times each day the patient noted on a diary sheet his body weight; intake and output of fluids; the number of aspirin taken; oral temperature; the time of onset, location, severity, and duration of joint stiffness and pain; and any changes in feeling of well-being. The patients were also asked to note any changes they observed, or thought they observed, in the "weather" in the chamber.

At the start of each patient's residence in the Climatron, all the climate factors were kept at a constant level. The patient was thus able to get adjusted to the room and the daily routine of examination and record keeping. Of course this uniform condition also gave the researchers a base for comparison with the patient's reactions to the "atmospheric changes" made later.

At the end of a five- to seven-day period, the doctors began manipulating the "climate" in the chamber. One procedure was to increase the atmospheric pressure over a two-hour period to 31.5—a reading the barometer would give in a period of fine, clear weather. Then, over a four-hour period, they brought the atmospheric pressure down to a low reading of 28.5 inches, representing a condition that would exist as a storm rapidly approached. The pressure would then be returned to the standard base of 30 inches. Pressure was the only change made in this phase of the test.

A day later a cycle of humidity changes was carried out, with the relative humidity being increased from the comfortable 30 percent to 80 percent, and then back down over a period of hours. Again, this was the only factor changed.

A day or two after that, air pressure and humidity were simultaneously put through changing cycles. That is, as the barometer fell, the humidity went up, or vice versa. In some experiments the cycles of change were slowed, so that for long periods of time, low barometer/high humidity—or other combinations—remained in effect for hours.

The carefully kept records showed the researchers exactly what kind of "weather" increased the miseries of arthritis patients. The falling atmospheric pressure teamed up with rising humidity to show "significant worsening of arthritis." Falling pressure or rising humidity alone did not account for the ill effects, nor did the exact level of either pressure or humidity. The real culprit was found to be the combined change in these two factors.

What About a Change of Climate?

People are afflicted with arthritis in every geographical area of the world—in the tropics, in the Arctic, in mild climates, and in stormy ones. But the evidence is plain, both from the Hollander research and from the observations of innumerable patients and their physicians, that some climates do increase suffering. The greatest suffering of weather-sensitive people occurs in climates like those of the upper midwestern and northeastern United States—along the storm track—where falling pressures and rising humidity are often present together.

If you keep a weather diary of your own, you will be able to tell whether you're being affected by this combination—or by other factors in the weather. Some arthritics are affected simply by continued high humidity in cold weather. Others find hot, humid weather harder to take. If you're an arthritis sufferer, there is a strong likelihood that you're being affected by the pressure-humidity factor, but it is possible that something else in the weather may be troubling you, too.

What kind of climate should you choose? There's not a single Sunbelt state, either humid or dry, that lacks boosters. After consulting with many arthritis victims and with many physicians, we believe that the best refuge for arthritis is a warm, stable, dry climate.

We must repeat that such a climate—in fact, any climate—will not provide a cure for your arthritis. It will only help to alleviate your painful symptoms. The Arthritis Foundation states, "There is no evidence that the disease itself changes or gets better in a warm, dry climate."

However, note that phrase "the disease itself." In that connection we'd like to quote an Arizona rheumatologist who says, "I think my colleagues are unduly reluctant to concede that if the symptoms are sufficiently alleviated it amounts to a cure—at least if the patient so perceives it. I don't want to sound like a chamber of commerce booster, but in my practice I have observed hundreds of cases in which there have been symptomatic remissions that to the patient seemed 'miraculous.' Whatever their clinical condition, these patients are far better off than they were in the climates where they formerly resided. Of course, I must admit, I've seen some cases where the patient was not helped at all, and I suppose if I were a northern physician today—as I once was—I would be hesitant about stating flatly to any of my patients that they should move forthwith to the Southwest desert and that all would then be well."

It is nevertheless undeniable that many arthritics fare well in the Southwest. Some cases we've garnered from physicians, and from patients themselves, are illustrative:

• A fifty-nine-year-old businessman from New York had suffered for fifteen years from rheumatoid arthritis. Within ten days of his arrival in Tucson he was able to walk freely, and his medication was reduced by half.

• A thirty-five-year-old rheumatoid arthritis sufferer had surgery to remove diseased tissue from a joint. He was in great pain after the surgery and moved from Illinois to New Mexico. The pain largely disappeared and he was able to go back to his profession as a laboratory technician. Neither he nor his doctor is sure that the remission is a result of climate or whether it should be attributed to successful surgery. However, on a visit to his former home he reported "considerable pain" in arthritic joints other than the surgical site.

• A fifty-one-year-old teacher with an eleven-year history of rheumatoid arthritis moved from Massachusetts to Nevada, where she was almost immediately able to discard her cane.

Although the odds seem to favor weather-sensitive arthritics who move to dry, warm climates, many arthritics have found relief in the warm but humid climates of the Gulf Coast, Florida, and other southeastern states. Possibly those who show a marked improvement in their arthritis symptoms in these areas are not true weather sensitives. Not all arthritics are.

Some victims of arthritis who move to high altitudes experience "dramatic remission" of their discomfort shortly after their arrival. Researchers trace this to "improvement in overall thermoregulation efficiency." Persons with certain forms of arthritis (as well as asthma and allergy victims) have deficiencies in those bodily mechanisms that regulate heat. Altitude seems to restore this mechanism to more normal operation.

15

Can Climate Help Your Heart?

There is no climate that will magically cure a coronary disease, but there are places that can help you feel better, and possibly even live longer, even if you have a serious heart problem. In the Sunbelt, and in other sections of the country, we have talked to heart patients who have found their afflictions easier to put up with because they made a move. We suspect there are a great many people who, if they had a better understanding of what weather, climate, and environment do to their hearts, could live healthier, more comfortable lives right where they are.

We've asked many physicians this question: "Do you feel that moving to a 'better' climate can benefit some heart patients?" Opinions are divided, as they are concerning moving because of any other disease. "A move can be definitely beneficial under some circumstances," said a Minnesota cardiologist. "I often advise my patients to move to a place that doesn't have such severe weather—especially such extremes of temperature—and some have certainly been helped by more benign climates."

Weather and Your Heart

Doctors and patients alike regard getting away from the cold as a definite gain, especially for angina sufferers. "Angina episodes are much more frequent in winter than during the warmer months," says a medical textbook. Angina patients are warned not to walk on cold days, especially facing wind. But even in still air simply going out into cold can trigger an attack.

Most angina patients who have relocated to warmer climates are glad they made the move. A middle-aged man in Florida told us that in his native Pennsylvania his doctor had advised him not to go outside on cold winter days without wearing a face mask. "He said that exposing any area of the skin to cold can bring on an angina episode. But I felt ridiculous going out in what seemed to most people like a moderate temperature— maybe just a little below freezing. There I was, all muffled up like it was twenty below. Of course I had to do it. I'm sure glad I don't have that problem anymore."

Cold in itself is a danger for heart patients, and the additional strain placed on the heart by going from a heated house into cold temperatures outdoors is often more than they should—or can—take. It results, as heart patients are frequently warned by their physicians, in a "marked rise in arterial blood pressure." The quick transition from a house at 70° F. to an outdoor temperature of, say, 20° F. may prove stimulating to a person with a normal heart, but that fifty-degree difference can cause acute discomfort and even danger for those with heart problems. This is a major consideration for physicians who advise some of their patients to seek a warmer climate.

Any heart patient must also regard heat—particularly humid heat—as a serious threat to his health and well-being. Dr. Herbert Austin, of the National Oceanic and Atmospheric Administration, reports that heart-disease emergencies are often 20 percent above the expected rate during heat waves.

A study of twelve heat waves in New York City showed increases in deaths of the elderly in general. The most marked increase was among those with heart disease. A National Institute of Health–sponsored study of thirty-two metropolitan areas containing 40 percent of the U.S. population revealed mortality to be consistently lowest among heart patients when air temperature was in the 60s and 70s; as the temperature went up, mortality rose sharply. However, in the Sunbelt cities of Miami, Tampa, Houston, and Phoenix, the lowest mortality was at temperatures between 80° F. and 89° F., no doubt because persons living in these warmer cities are acclimated to the heat.

Other studies indicate that excessive heat may play a role in susceptibility to hypertensive heart disease. This conclusion is drawn from a study in Tecumseh, Michigan, where it was found that persons who had suffered heat stroke in the past were five times more likely to develop heart trouble later in life than those who had no previous history of heart illness. Such observations, report researchers F. P. Ellis of the University of Birmingham, England, and Freida Nelson of the Health Department of New York City, "suggest the need for careful assessment of the possibly aggravating effects of climatic factors in intensifying the course of hypertensive disease."

A biometeorologist who has been called the world's foremost authority on how climate affects heart disease is Dr. George Burch of the Department of Medicine, Tulane University. In his practice at Charity Hospital in New Orleans, this eminent cardiologist has frequently observed the rise in admissions to the hospital under certain weather conditions. The increase was always greatest among patients with heart disease, the aged, the debilitated, and those with cerebrovascular accidents.

Not content with merely observing, Dr. Burch set out to conduct a set of tests that he hoped would show exactly the clinical effects of a warm, humid atmosphere on patients with congestive heart failure. To do that he set up a hospital room as a climate chamber in which temperature, humidity, and air movement could be controlled. He observed a number of patients under a variety of "weather" conditions over a long period of time. Some remained in the room for two days, some for as long as sixteen days. Temperatures tried ranged from a neutral level of 75° F. with a relative humidity of 41 percent, to 95° F. with a relative humidity as high as 81 percent.

Dr. Burch reported that "the majority of patients with CHF

[congestive heart failure] developed symptoms of distress at the higher temperature and humidity levels, but in all instances the symptoms disappeared almost immediately after the room conditions were returned to normal." Further, he reported, "All subjects found the warm, humid environment unpleasant and became restless or complained as time elapsed."

Air Pollution and Your Heart

There is a factor in the environment that is far more dangerous to the health of coronary-disease sufferers than anything in the weather. That is air pollution. While it's bad for all of us, it can be disastrous for anyone in poor health, particularly for the victims of heart disease. In particular, carbon monoxide places a severe strain on the heart—anybody's heart—with far worse effects on those with any heart impairment.

Carbon monoxide "crowds out" the oxygen the body needs. Studies have shown that even in healthy persons, exposure to carbon monoxide in quantities often found in urban air "may be followed by disturbances of the cardiac rhythm." The disturbances are far greater in heart patients.

While there are other factors in urban living that place a strain on the heart—stress, for instance—the American Lung Association states that mortality figures clearly reveal the effect of air pollution on health: "Death rates for coronary heart disease are 37 percent higher for men and 46 percent higher for women in metropolitan areas," reports the association. "An Illinois study found cardiovascular death rates more than 25 percent higher for male Chicagoans between the ages of 25 and 35 than for their counterparts in rural areas. The difference was *100 percent* for men between 35 and 45 and nearly *200 percent* for men between 55 and 64." (The italics are ours.)

Numerous studies show a direct relationship between high levels of air pollution and deaths among those with chronic heart disease. In Los Angeles, hospital admissions for 223 consecutive days were studied and correlated with air-pollution levels. The direct relationship to carbon monoxide was clearly demonstrated. Less extensive studies in other cities show the same linking of high carbon monoxide ratings to increased hospital admissions and higher death rates for coronary patients.

A report by Drs. John R. Goldsmith of California's Department of Health and Wilbert S. Aronow of the University of California College of Medicine at Irvine concludes that there are five ways in which carbon monoxide can affect cardiac function or coronary disease:

1. Aggravation of angina pectoris. This occurs after exposure to 50 ppm of CO after ninety minutes.
2. Aggravation of intermittent spasm of the arteries. This occurs after exposure to 50 ppm of CO for two hours.
3. Alteration of the electrocardiogram in normal subjects. This probably will occur following exposure to 100 ppm of CO after four hours of exposure. (This effect has also been observed in certain occupations where exposure to CO is high, such as fire fighting.)
4. Production or aggravation of atherosclerosis associated with carbon monoxide in smoking.
5. Impairment of survival in patients with acute myocardial infarction.

Drs. Goldsmith and Aronow feel the evidence for the last two points is suggestive and that for the first three points convincing.

We have talked to people with coronary problems in rural areas and small towns who have heeded the advice frequently given by physicians aware of the effects of air pollution: "Move out of the city." Even without a doctor's telling them so, many have recognized these effects for themselves.

In his book *Breathing for Survival*, Casimir Nikel gives a vivid account of what made him move from a large Ohio city to a small one in New Mexico: "I noticed that when I was driving in congested traffic, the fumes from autos in front of me, particularly during a waiting period at a traffic light, would precipitate chest pains. Finally while walking only one block from the hospital at which I was employed to a nearby bank, I suffered a severe onset of angina pain. By this time my heart was beset by several serious symptoms: tachycardia, arrhythmia, limited cardiac reserve, and extremely slow recovery. Even moderate exertion would require several hours for my heart to return to the generally acceptable normal pulse of eighty beats per minute. Because the temperature outdoors was mild, but the automotive smog was heavy that memorable March 29, I assumed that I was in extreme danger in that metropolis. It was then that I decided that a move was imperative for me. I must say, however, that I had not the slightest perception of what new knowledge this decision would lead me to."

If you are considering moving for health reasons, but can't quite bring yourself to face up to all the problems ahead and all the advantages you will have to leave behind, consider Nikel's position. He had been with the same hospital for twenty-one years, the last five of them serving as its chief administrator. His hospital was expanding. He stood a chance of being promoted to the position of an executive director.

"But," says Nikel, "that last angina attack said to me, 'Either stay for all these marvelous professional challenges or leave and maybe extend your crippled health for a few scanty years.' "

Nikel accomplished a lot more than that. Soon after moving he was able to discontinue his peritrate and nitroglycerine medication, and some four months after his arrival in the Southwest he had an experience that dramatized the improvement in his health. Touring Carlsbad Caverns, he walked down to the lowest level, only to find that he had gone considerably below the depth to which the elevator descended.

"This forced me," he relates, "to walk 77 feet up extremely steep ramps. This I negotiated with only one rest stop. Only a year before I was unable to negotiate two flights of stairs without taking a nitroglycerine pill to stop my angina pectoris pains." Years later, Nikel was able to report that "all symptoms of tachychardia, arrhythmia and limited cardiac reserve" had disappeared.

Was his remarkable recovery due to the salubrious climate to which he had moved? It certainly helped, Nikel will admit, but he attributes most of his improvement to the fact that he escaped from the pollution in the city in which he formerly lived—a city where the air was leading to his "slow suffocation."

Altitude and Your Heart

Among the millions who are thinking about either moving to or visiting the mountain West are many people with some kind of coronary problem. If you are one of them, you may well ask the question that confronts many physicians: "Is it all right for me to go to a high altitude, or will it be hard on my heart?"

If you're talking about climbing to peaks over 10,000 feet—don't. But if you're thinking about the mile-high altitudes of cities such as Denver, Colorado Springs, or Albuquerque, medicine can give you reassuring answers.

We have often had friends from back East express doubts about the advisability of their coming to visit us at our 7,000-foot New Mexico location. However, one adventurous friend from New Jersey, a woman in her fifties, who had had heart trouble for years and who had undergone a triple bypass operation about a year and a half earlier, came without trepidation and even drove with us to the top of our nearby mountain, almost 11,000 feet high. At that height she went for a short hike, suffering no symptoms whatsoever.

In a test conducted by University of Colorado researchers, the reactions of patients with known coronary disease to high altitudes were compared with those of healthy subjects who had no detectable heart ailments. Involved in the test were eleven male patients, seven who had suffered myocardial infarctions, two with angina, and two who had past myocardial infarctions and also had angina. They were successively tested, while active, at altitudes of 5,200, 8,000, and 10,400 feet. The researchers reported that there was "no significant difference" between the performance of the hearts of the coronary patients and that of the healthy controls. This particular test is typical of many similar ones that have yielded the same results.

Some doctors do express doubts about the wisdom of heart patients going to much higher altitudes—such as the top of Pikes Peak, which is 14,110 feet high—but others see no danger in such excursions. Most caution that anyone with a known heart condition should at least stop a few days at a Denver-high altitude before venturing higher. Others simply advise that if any untoward symptoms are observed—pounding heart, erratic heartbeat, shortness of breath, feeling of faintness, chest pain—a person should return to a lower altitude as soon as possible, where, almost invariably, the symptoms will promptly go away. Certainly anyone with a heart condition, or a history of heart trouble, should seek medical advice before moving to, or vacationing in, any high-altitude area.

Should You Move?

The first and most fundamental piece of advice to anybody with any ailment at all is *consult your physician*. That, of course, is doubly important advice for people suffering with any form of coronary disease.

The circumstances that should be considered which might make your life more comfortable, if not longer, are:

Weather. You may find that you'll be healthier if the place you move to is less subject to extreme heat or cold. If you now live where it gets either very hot or very cold, or both, don't subject yourself to sudden temperature changes by going out into the cold from a heated house or out into the heat from an air-conditioned one any more than you have to.

Air pollution. The carbon monoxide spewed into urban air by automobiles can have serious ill effects for heart patients. It may be better for you to move to a suburb, small town, or rural area. If that isn't possible, consider moving to a section of your present city where there is less pollution. In general, the larger the city, the more automobiles and the more carbon monoxide pollution.

Altitude. No problem here at moderate mile-high altitudes, but check with your physician about altitudes higher than that.

16

How to Pick the Right Climate for You

Anyone considering moving for health reasons would, ideally, have the opportunity to live in many sections of the country. Finding and choosing a new place to live isn't easy. Many people make mistakes in doing it. They fail to get enough advance information about the place they move to; they neglect to take into consideration all the factors to which thought must be given; and, perhaps worst of all, they choose a new climate without making sure that it's really the kind of climate in which they want to, or should, be living.

Pulling up your roots from one place and, without damaging them too much, trying to transplant them to another soil requires a considerable amount of both money and energy. You may not be able to afford it, in terms of either coin, more than once. So it is of the utmost importance that you choose wisely and well. Moving to the Ozarks because Uncle Joe says, "It's great," or to Colorado because some former neighbors "have done very well there," is no reason whatsoever for you to feel that either of these places might be right for you.

Before deciding to move, you should be aware of how your health is either related to, or made worse by, the climate or the environment in which you live, and of *exactly* what factors are troubling you.

Chart Your Own Weather Reactions

The science of biometeorology has not yet progressed to the stage where you can go to an institution or specialist for a test that will give you the answers to your own personal questions about what climate and weather are doing to *you*. Of course, it is possible that you already know—maybe all too well. But if you've simply had some rather vague thoughts that there is some link between your bad days and what it's doing outside but have never quite figured out just what they are, you should set out to practice some do-it-yourself biometerology in a serious effort to find out.

The best way to do that is to keep your own personal weather record. In it you should enter, every day for a specified period, observations about your physical and mental condition, along with a record of temperatures, barometric pressures, relative humidity readings, and, perhaps, data such as sky conditions, wind directions and velocities, and air pollution. You won't be able to keep a record of the numbers and kinds of ions in the air. Such readings are just not available from the usual weather information sources, nor is there an inexpensive instrument that will enable you to make your own readings.

Ideally, you would keep such a weather record over a long enough period to tell you how you react to these weather phenomena in all seasons. Or you could keep such a record for one month in each season—the first month in each season, preferably, because then your body is making adjustments to new meteorological conditions, and how you react to seasonal changes is highly significant.

Your record can consist of simple notations on a calendar or in a notebook, but it will probably tell you a lot more if you keep it in the form of a chart, such as the one shown on the next page. The entries describing your personal feelings, physical and men-

SUGGESTED PERSONAL WEATHER REACTION CHART

		Temperature	Humidity	Barometer	Clear/Cloudy	Wind	Physical Reactions	Psychological Reactions
Sunday	Morning Afternoon Evening							
Monday	Morning Afternoon Evening							
Tuesday	Morning Afternoon Evening							
Wednesday	Morning Afternoon Evening							
Thursday	Morning Afternoon Evening							
Friday	Morning Afternoon Evening							
Saturday	Morning Afternoon Evening							

tal, can be as simple or as elaborate as you want to make them. It all depends on how sharply you're trying to define and understand your own weather reactions.

You can obtain your data from TV weathercasts, the daily newspaper, calls to the weather service, or by reading your own weather instruments, which are purchasable.

Whether your personal weather response record is extensive or limited, you can expect to reap rich benefits from keeping it. Knowing if the weather is affecting you and just what factors in the weather are doing it will give you the vital information you need to make a decision as to whether you should stay where you are or think about moving.

Get Information about Climates

If you decide to embark on a search for a better climate—that is, a better climate for *you*—you should learn as much as you can about possible places. Books and magazine articles will give you some information, though often it is too vague. The best source for climate information is a government agency associated with the National Weather Service—the National Climatic Center. This agency dispenses climate data in understandable, usable form. In addition to answering individual queries about climate from citizens—a lot of doctors among them—the center puts out a number of publications.

Its *Local Climatological Data* bulletins present, in great detail, information about the weather in some 300 U.S. communities. Among them are all the major cities in the Sunbelt, as well as many smaller ones. You can get a free list of communities on which climate data have been prepared by writing to the National Climatic Center, Federal Building, Asheville, North Carolina 28801.

For any one of the communities on which the center has prepared data you can purchase reports. You can obtain a report about the weather in any given month for 20 cents, or an annual report for the same price. You can, if you wish, subscribe to the reports on a given community; for $2.55 you will get the twelve monthly reports and the annual report. (An order must be for at least $2.)

Both monthly and annual reports give you facts about:

Temperature, including the high and low recorded at a particular instrument location in the community; the average highest and lowest temperatures for a thirty-year period; the averages of all daily temperatures for the thirty-year period.

Precipitation, including average precipitation for each month during a thirty-year period; the greatest and least amounts recorded in any one month; the most that fell in any one day; the forms of precipitation—rain, snow, ice, or sleet.

Humidity, including the average relative humidities at midnight, 6 A.M., 12 noon, and 6 P.M.

Wind, including average speeds of wind in miles per hour by day and month; direction of wind; highest wind speeds recorded.

Sunshine, giving figures about the percentage of possible sunlight received.

Cloudiness, giving the number of days with various amounts of cloud cover.

Studying the reports and comparing the data about one community with data from others will reveal fascinating, and surprising, facts. For instance . . .

· Asheville, North Carolina, in the Great Smoky Mountains, which you might expect to be dry, is more humid than New Orleans in the summer. Morning relative humidity in Asheville in July is 97 percent, while in "steaming" New Orleans it's 84 percent.

· Miami gets 72 percent of the possible sunlight in February; Tampa receives 67 percent.

· California cities show astonishing differences in percentage of possible sunlight. January figures show Sacramento with 45 percent, San Francisco with 56 percent, San Diego with 68 percent.

· Houston gets 46 inches of rainfall annually, while Brownsville, not very far down the Gulf Coast, gets only 27 inches.

• Mile-high Denver has an average high temperature for July of 88° F., while Charleston, South Carolina, has an average July high only one degree higher, at 89. Of course, the nighttime lows are a different story. In Charleston, the thermometer goes down to 72 (July average), but in Denver it drops to 57.

The chamber of commerce in almost any community will be glad to send you literature. Some of the brochures from C of Cs contain valuable climatic and environmental information, but they're often incomplete and, of course, likely to be biased. The information is not necessarily false, but will be presented so as to put the community in the best light.

After you've narrowed down your choice of a place to live, you will of course want to make a visit there. Ideally you'd make several visits.

Visit Phoenix in January when blizzards are howling across the North and you might well think this sunny climate is just the place for you. But go there again in midsummer, with the thermometer pushing 110 in the shade, and even though the humidity may be down there at 10 percent, you might be repelled by the sheer heat. Such a visit could prompt you to look elsewhere, to think about some other location in the Southwest or in California—someplace that may be equally dry, but where it doesn't get that hot. Like nearby Tucson, which is somewhat cooler; or El Paso, Texas; or some smaller communities in southern New Mexico; or not quite so dry, but still comfortable, San Diego County.

Try visiting possible Florida choices in September, a miserable month when the heat is a wet blanket and hurricanes sometimes threaten, and you might well wonder if you really want to live *there* all year round.

Retired persons are fortunate in that they have time and can, finances permitting, make their visits longer than the standard two- or three-week vacation. Staying as long as possible is especially important if you're trying out a radically new climate, one you've never experienced before. If you make a winter visit to

Florida or California's low desert, or any other really warm location, and have come from below-freezing temperatures in the North, it takes your body a while to get adjusted to temperatures in the 70s, 80s, or maybe even 90s. It's not a fair test to make too brief a visit. You may feel better during that time than you would if you lived there all the time—then again you may not feel as good.

If you're checking out a high-altitude place in a western mountain state, your early reactions might be unfavorable. You may experience fatigue, dizziness, and a feeling of malaise for the first few days—sometimes the first weeks—at high altitudes. So a short stay can give you a very distorted picture.

While you're visiting any community, your most valuable source of information about it is the people who live there. Talk to them, ask them questions. You'll find most people like to talk about the places they live. Don't rely on real-estate people or others with any vested interest in getting you to stay there. Strike up conversations with people in stores, on buses, sitting on benches. Retirees are usually eager to share their thoughts about the place to which they have retired. From them you'll get an impartial catalog of both its virtues and drawbacks. If you visit any Senior Citizens Center you'll find scores of individuals who are more than willing to express their opinions. Many retired persons have done a lot of traveling and can give you information about other places, too.

If your stay is long enough—if it lasts beyond the initial period of adjustment—you would do well to keep up your weather diary. Just as it told you a lot about your reactions to the weather back home, it will tell you how you respond to this new, and possibly strange, place.

You should keep in mind that your reactions are probably somewhat colored by the excitement of what you are seeing, doing, and experiencing, and by the fact that you are on vacation. You have left many of your troubles behind you. You aren't coping with all of the domestic, interpersonal, family—and possibly work—problems that go with everyday living at home.

Some Things to Think About

The act of moving isn't a simple one. It disrupts your way of life, the routines you're used to, your familiar forms of recreation. It can result in the breaking up of meaningful friendships and can take you away from family members and other relatives whom you may not have realized you needed—or even cared that much about—until you are away from them. It's all too easy to gloss over these matters with some such thought as, "Oh, well, it's only a three-hour jet flight away," but how many times a year are you going to be able to make that flight back home?

Homesickness. No matter what the improvement in climate and no matter how much better your health is, if you continue to feel like a displaced person in an alien land, if you have left your heart elsewhere, you don't stand a very good chance of improving your lot.

Everyone who moves feels, at some time or other, homesick for what was left behind. Psychologists have found this to be the case even when conditions in the former place of residence were very uncomfortable. People can even get nostalgic about acquaintances they disliked and the stench of garbage-littered streets. But the kind of homesickness we are referring to is the awful ache in the solar plexus that never leaves, the panicky feeling in the stomach and head that makes you want to rush back to whatever it was you once had.

The first question to try to settle in your mind is, "Can I move at all or am I really tied to where I am?" Once having made a move, even though you find yourself unhappy, it's not all that easy to go back.

Seasonal patterns. One of the things that can increase your homesickness is a move to a part of the country that has seasonal patterns different from those of the region in which you had previously lived. Many northerners who have moved to the Sunbelt find themselves uncomforable about the lack of distinctively different seasons of the year. Some typical complaints include: "Monotonous" . . . "Too much of a good thing" . . . "There's nothing to look forward to." Other feelings are harder to put into words, consisting as they do of vague stirrings of discontent.

This is more than a psychological matter; it's a physiological one as well. If you've always lived where there is a hot summer and a cold winter and clearly defined springs and falls in between, your body may be so tuned to these cycles that it will have a hard time adjusting to a climate that does not have marked changes between one season and another.

Unfamiliarity can create anxiety. There can be factors in any new place that, largely because they are unfamiliar to you, might unduly upset your state of mind. We talked to a retired couple in Texas who became extremely anxious every time it rained a few inches because they had learned that once, years ago, the town they had selected for retirement had suffered a serious flood. The woman had developed ulcers since their move and the man's heart condition was actually worse, although he had expected it to become better. Naturally, they were beginning to wonder if their move from Minneapolis had been worth it.

We spoke to a man in California who was so worried about a possible earthquake that he was considering moving back to his home in the East. His asthma, he said, hadn't been helped all that much anyway, and now his doctor was having to prescribe tranquilizers for him so that he could sleep.

In Pensacola we spoke to a woman who said that as soon as the hurricane season approached she was a "nervous wreck." Her anxieties had become so great that she was making plans to move back to Wisconsin. In that state she had actually witnessed two devastating tornadoes, one of which had blown away the barn on the farm on which she had grown up. When we asked her if she didn't feel the same kind of fear there, her answer was, "Oh, no, I was used to tornadoes." None of the arguments we tried to muster about how tornadoes give you little warning, if any, but that you have plenty of time to run from the path of a hurricane, meant anything at all to her. It was a purely unreasoning fear over which she had no control.

Country living stress. The United States seems to be in a "let's move to the country" phase, with increasing numbers of Americans dreaming of a few acres somewhere away from the hustle and bustle, the noise and pollution, the stresses and strains of the city. If you are one of them, wait a minute; there are problems in country living, too.

Elizabeth Forsberg, M.D., a Vermont psychiatrist, in speaking of former city dwellers who have moved to her state, says, "You see the signs—the headaches, the stomach aches, the heart palpitations, the incredible stress. It settles in the muscles and creates all types of physical problems."

Families who move to the country because they think it will provide a better way of life for the children are often surprised to find the kids hate it; feeding chickens and cleaning rabbit hutches was never *their* idea of a good time. People who are commuting to jobs in the city find it more of a strain than they had expected it would be and the long list of things to do "while you're there in town" often creates conflicts.

For those who are retired, the long drives to stores, to doctors' offices, and to visit friends can be particularly burdensome. And for anybody the unexpected can sometimes turn what was hoped would be a peaceful life-style into one seemingly never-ending round of emergencies. The car won't start, the pump breaks down, the power goes off, the road washes out, the grasshoppers eat the garden down to the ground, the washing machine goes on the blink and the repairman "can't get out to your area until next week."

Country living, which you envision as a more economical way of life, can turn out to be a lot more expensive. Country families, for example, spend 42 percent more for gasoline.

If you seriously think of moving to the country, whether to a place close to where you now live or to some garden spot in a totally different part of the country, you would do well to buy the U.S. Department of Agriculture's 472-page book *Living on a Few Acres,* which has in it such pertinent chapters as "Consider the Tradeoffs Before Leaving the City." (Send $7 to Superintendent of Documents, U.S. Government Printing Office, Washington, D.C. 20402.)

Other family members. If you are not yet of retirement age, or at least of an age where you no longer have other family members to consider—if there is such an age—you should not try to make any unilateral decisions about moving to a new place, especially if it's someplace distant from where you now live. Children—particularly teenagers—often take very unkindly to moving at all. We've heard of cases in which they have reacted very badly, even when the move was considered to be a lifesaving one for a parent. One unhappy mother told us of their experience in moving to Florida for her husband's health. "Our son—he's only sixteen—came with us, but he wouldn't stay. He went back to Indiana to live with his older brother."

Even spouses who go along with a move with apparent enthusiasm, or at least compliance, can harbor feelings of hostility toward their partners for having been expected to give up a familiar city, home, associations with relatives, jobs, or way of life. We ran into at least one divorce that resulted from a move that hadn't been clearly talked out. So be sure you do discuss the proposed move—backwards, forwards, and sideways—and make certain that all involved parties are in agreement about it. Often family members can come to accept a move if they feel they have had plenty of say in it and enough time to get adjusted to it, and that nobody has put one over on them. Also—there are lots of places. If you can't agree on one, maybe you can agree on another.

Economics. Nobody can be happy—or healthy—anywhere if his income does not support his life-style. If you are retired and on a fixed income, make sure that any place you're thinking of moving to isn't more expensive than the place you now live, or that you can afford it if it is. If you need to supplement your retirement income, check out the possibilities for doing so in the new location. If you are still of working age, moving may be much more difficult. It isn't easy to leave a position in which you have developed some seniority, or to start out again in a new job. Of course, if you are young and just starting out—the world is your oyster: any place may be a possible place in which to live.

When Dr. Merril Eisenbud, director of New York University's Laboratory for Environmental Science, was asked, "With all the pollution, where in the world is the healthiest place to live?" he answered without hesitation, "Where you have a job."

He added that all the things that go with economic security—good food, good housing, and other favorable qualities of life—help to make life healthful. In his opinion, economic stability, and all that it implies, is actually a more important consideration than the dangers of air pollution.

The Medical Aspects of Moving

Whether you're moving because you already have some medical problem that you feel might be helped by a change or because you just want to stay healthy and feel that a better climate might help you do that, it is important that you think about the medical aspects of leaving one place and going to make your home in another.

If you have been under medical care, talk to your doctor about your plans. You may find that he or she doesn't know too much about climates or biometeorology, but then again, you may be fortunate enough to have a doctor who is interested in the subject of how climate affects health; an increasing number of physicians are.

Once you are established in your new community, don't wait for an emergency to arise before you find a doctor. The county medical society, or a nearby medical school, can recommend family physicians or specialists. At the local library you can consult the *American Medical Directory*, which lists every medical doctor in the United States and gives his age and medical school attended. It also tells whether a doctor is a member of the AMA and whether he or she has held any faculty posts. Specialists are listed as "Board Certified" if they have chosen to take a special examination and have passed. Not all doctors take the examination, and the fact that they haven't doesn't mean they are not qualified. Those doctors who have not taken the exam but who have the training and background to practice in their specialty are rated as "Board Eligible."

Of course, you are hardly going to pick a doctor because he went to a certain school, or because he's a certain age, or because you like his or her name. So lists have their limits. Here, again, it is wise to talk to people—particularly persons in your own age bracket, or with the same ailments that are plaguing you. They can tell you much about a doctor's manner, personality, fees, availability, apparent caring, whether or not he takes kindly to questions over the telephone, and so forth.

Be sure you speak to your new doctor about any possible changes that should be made in medications you take. As you will recall from the chapters on heat and cold, temperature has a bearing on the dosage of many prescription drugs. Even if you are just going to a different climate for an extended visit, you should talk to your doctor at home about this matter.

In a new location, you'll probably be much more conscious of how you are feeling simply because you'll be watching for signs that you are either better or worse. This can have both its advantages and its perils. On the one hand, you may tend to exaggerate ills that went unnoticed back home. Then again, you may lay the emphasis on your feelings of well-being. That, of course, would be all to the good. Even if any improvement you believe you have noticed doesn't show up in clinical tests, even if you baffle your doctor, if you *think* you are better in a certain place, that can be the first step toward your actually *being* better.

You may well have found where to live for your health.

Appendix

National
Climatic Center
Sample Data

To provide a picture of the comprehensive nature of the National Climatic Center's Annual Summaries, we reprint, on the following pages, the data from a sample Annual Summary.

Local Climatological Data—1978

Asheville, North Carolina

NARRATIVE CLIMATOLOGICAL SUMMARY

The city of Asheville is located on both banks of the French Broad River, near the center of the French Broad Basin. Upstream from Asheville, the valley runs south for 18 miles and then curves toward the south-southwest; downstream from the City, the valley is oriented toward the north-northwest. Two miles upstream from the principal section of Asheville, the Swannanoa River joints the French Broad from the east. The entire valley is known as the "Asheville Plateau," having an average elevation near 2,200 feet above mean sea level, and is flanked by mountain ridges to the east and west, whose peaks range from 2,000 to 4,400 feet above the valley floor. At the Carolina-

Tennessee border, about 25 miles north-northwest of Asheville, a relatively high ridge of mountains blocks the northern end of the valley. Thirty miles south, the Blue Ridge Mountains form an escarpment, having a general elevation of about 2,700 feet m.s.l. The tallest peaks near Asheville are Mt. Mitchell, 6,684 feet m.s.l., 20 miles northeast of the City, and Big Pisgah Mountain, 5,721 feet m.s.l., 16 miles to the southwest.

Asheville has a temperate, but invigorating climate. Considerable variation in temperature often occurs from day to day in summer, as well as during the other seasons. Temperature extremes at the City Office ranging from −7° to 99° have been recorded during the last 34 years of record, ending with 1964. The National Weather Service Office was located at the Asheville Airport on September 1, 1964. The warmest day of record, with an average temperature of 85°, was June 27, 1952, with a maximum temperature of 97°, and a minimum reading of 72°. The coldest day of record at the City Office, with an average temperature of 3°, was February 5, 1917, with a maximum temperature of 9°, and a minimum reading of −4°. Airport records indicate January 30, 1966, as the coldest day of record there with an average temperature of 2° as derived from a maximum of 11° and a minimum of −7°.

While the office was located in the City, the combination of roof exposure conditions and a smoke blanket, caused by inversions in temperature in the valley on quiet nights, resulted in higher early morning temperatures at City Office sites than were experienced nearer ground level in nearby rural areas. The growing season in this area is of sufficient length for commercial crops, the average length of freeze-free period being 195 days, based on City Office data. The average data of last occurrence in spring of a temperature 32° or lower is April 12; of 28°, March 29; of 20°, February 27. The average date of first occurrence in fall of 32° is October 24; of 28°, November 4; of 20°, December 4.

The orientation of the French Broad Valley appears to have a pronounced influence on the wind direction; prevailing winds are from the northwest during all months of the year. Also, the shielding effect of the nearby mountain barriers apparently has a direct bearing on the annual amount of precipitation received in this vicinity. Within the area roughly bounded by a line connecting Asheville, Weaverville, Marshall, Leicester, and Enka, the average annual precipitation is 38 inches, the lowest in North Carolina. Precipitation increases somewhat to the northwest of the Asheville-Marshall-Enka area and increases sharply in all other directions, especially to the south and southwest, where the average annual precipitation becomes more than 60 inches within 30 miles of Asheviille.

Destructive events caused directly by meteorological conditions are infrequent. The most frequent, occurring approximately at 12-year intervals, are floods on the French Broad River. These floods are usually associated with heavy rains from decelerating tropical storms moving over or near this area. The outstanding floods since the beginning of records are: July 16, 1916; August 16, 1928; August 13 and 30, 1940, September 29 and October 4–5, 1964; and November 5–6, 1977. According to historical records, destructive floods also occurred in April 1791; August 1796 and 1810; May 1845; August 1850 and 1852; and June 1876. Snowstorms which have seriously disrupted normal life in this community occurred on January 26, 1906; March 18, 1936; March 2–3, 1942, and repeated heavy snows in March 1960. Only one hailstorm of record caused considerable property damage in Asheville, that of June 18, 1936.

METEOROLOGICAL DATA FOR 1978

Station: Asheville, North Carolina—Asheville Airport.
Standard time used: Eastern.
Latitude: 35° 26′ N. Longitude: 82° 33′ W.
Elevation (ground): 2140 feet.

Month	Temperature °F							Degree days Base 65 °F		Precipitation in inches						Relative humidity, pct.			
	Averages			Extremes						Water equivalent			Snow, Ice pellets			Hour 01	Hour 07	Hour 13	Hour 19
	Daily maximum	Daily minimum	Monthly	Highest	Date	Lowest	Date	Heating	Cooling	Total	Greatest in 24 hrs.	Date	Total	Greatest in 24 hrs.	Date	(Local time)			
JAN	39.1	19.4	29.3	56	8	3	10	1101	0	7.47	2.95	24-25	9.7	3.0	19-20	82	87	65	73
FEB	44.2	22.5	33.4	68	25	6	7	878	0	0.44	0.18	13	5.3	3.7	21	74	83	56	62
MAR	58.9	32.8	45.9	78	31	14	5	586	0	5.22	1.77	9-10	5.3	4.2	2-3	82	87	51	60
APR	70.8	42.8	56.8	84	2	32	22	241	2	2.97	1.52	25-26	T	T	21	77	81	48	52
MAY	73.3	50.7	62.0	85	20	34	3	139	53	4.65	0.97	7-8	0.0	0.0		92	94	63	71
JUN	83.3	58.9	71.1	94	28	48	5	0	188	2.29	1.11	6-7	0.0	0.0		96	96	58	69
JUL	84.7	62.0	73.4	90	30	56	17	0	266	0.63	0.23	2	0.0	0.0		97	99	64	73
AUG	83.8	64.3	74.1	89	25	61	24	0	292	6.91	3.19	6-7	0.0	0.0		98	99	71	85
SEP	80.2	59.8	70.0	90	9	51	28	12	168	2.57	2.20	13-14	0.0	0.0		98	99	67	83
OCT	70.8	40.5	55.7	80	26	29	18	283	4	0.30	0.23	30-1	0.0	0.0		91	94	49	66
NOV	63.8	39.7	51.8	78	5	31	5	390	0	2.49	1.31	10	0.0	0.0		91	95	61	72
DEC	53.4	28.5	41.0	69	8	14	15	741	0	4.32	1.45	3-4	T	T	9	83	89	59	69
YEAR	67.2	43.5	55.4	94	JUN 28	3	JAN 10	4371	973	40.26	3.19	6-7	20.3	4.2	AUG 2-3	MAR	88	92	59	70

Month	Wind								Number of days											Average station pressure mb
	Resultant		Average speed m.p.h.	Fastest mile			Percent of possible sunshine	Average sky cover, tenths, sunrise to sunset	Sunrise to sunset			Precipitation .01 inch or more	Snow, Ice pellets 1.0 inch or more	Thunderstorms	Heavy fog, visibility ¼ mile or less.	Temperature °F				Elev. 2170 feet m.s.l.
	Direction	Speed m.p.h.		Speed m.p.h.	Direction	Date			Clear	Partly cloudy	Cloudy					Maximum		Minimum		
																90° and above (b)	32° and below	32° and below	0° and below	
JAN	34	6.1	11.1	32	34	9	47	6.1	11	5	15	13	4	1	8	0	6	28	0	940.1
FEB	33	5.0	9.6	31	33	22	56	6.0	6	11	11	5	1	0	2	0	2	25	0	939.7
MAR	33	2.7	9.5	31	35	10	61	5.8	10	7	14	15	1	3	2	0	2	12	0	940.1
APR	32	2.4	9.0	28	18	6	75	5.8	7	13	10	9	0	4	2	0	0	1	0	939.4
MAY	32	1.9	6.7	20	32	5	55	6.2	8	9	14	11	0	5	10	0	0	0	0	939.4
JUN	34	1.6	5.6	21	29	6	69	4.9	10	15	5	9	0	5	5	5	0	0	0	943.8
JUL	32	0.8	5.9	23	30	8	57	5.9	6	17	8	9	0	8	9	4	0	0	0	942.8
AUG	19	0.1	5.2	20	16	30	48	6.4	6	12	13	12	0	12	17	0	0	0	0	944.5
SEP	04	0.3	4.9	17	21	18	52	6.2	6	11	13	10	0	4	13	1	0	0	0	944.1
OCT	33	2.2	6.4	25	35	14	82	2.6	21	9	1	2	0	0	10	0	0	4	0	943.8
NOV	32	0.7	6.6	23	35	28	50	6.1	8	10	12	6	0	0	4	0	0	3	0	944.1
DEC	33	2.4	8.5	36	34	9	56	4.8	13	7	11	10	0	0	3	0	0	24	0	942.4
YEAR	33	2.1	7.4	36	34	DEC 9	59	5.6	112	126	127	111	6	42	85	10	10	97	0	942.0

NORMALS, MEANS, AND EXTREMES

	Temperatures °F							Normal Degree days Base 65 °F		Precipitation in inches										
	Normal			Extremes						Water equivalent							Snow, Ice pellets			
	Daily maximum	Daily minimum	Monthly	Record highest	Year	Record lowest	Year	Heating	Cooling	Normal	Maximum monthly	Year	Minimum monthly	Year	Maximum in 24 hrs.	Year	Maximum monthly	Year	Maximum in 24 hrs.	Year
				14		14					14		14		14		14		14	
	48.4	27.3	37.9	78	1975	-7	1966	840	0	3.39	7.47	1978	1.75	1970	2.95	1978	17.6	1966	7.6	1964
	50.6	28.2	39.4	77	1977	-2	1967	717	0	3.60	6.56	1966	0.44	1978	3.17	1966	25.5	1969	11.7	1969
	58.3	33.5	45.9	82	1974	14	1978	592	0	4.66	9.86	1975	2.59	1966	5.13	1968	13.0	1969	10.9	1969
	69.4	42.4	55.9	89	1972	24	1973	279	6	3.53	5.71	1973	0.25	1970	3.06	1973	0.2	1971	0.2	1971
	76.8	50.6	63.7	91	1969	29	1971	100	60	3.31	8.83	1973	1.72	1970	4.95	1973	0.0		0.0	
	82.5	58.7	70.6	96	1969	35	1966	14	182	3.97	6.54	1972	2.12	1975	3.54	1972	0.0		0.0	
	84.3	62.0	73.5	95	1970	46	1967	0	264	4.87	7.53	1969	0.63	1978	4.02	1969	0.0		0.0	
	83.8	61.8	72.8	94	1968	43	1968	0	244	4.50	11.28	1967	1.88	1972	4.12	1967	0.0		0.0	
	78.0	55.4	66.7	92	1975	30	1967	50	101	3.57	9.12	1977	1.17	1970	3.41	1975	0.0		0.0	
	69.1	44.5	56.8	84	1971	21	1976	269	15	3.25	7.05	1971	0.30	1978	2.95	1977	T	1977	T	1977
	58.2	34.3	46.3	81	1974	8	1970	561	0	2.94	6.88	1977	1.30	1965	4.03	1977	9.6	1968	5.7	1968
	49.3	28.1	38.7	78	1971	5	1977	815	0	3.59	8.48	1973	0.16	1965	2.66	1973	16.3	1971	16.3	1971
	67.4	44.0	55.7	96	JUN 1969	-7	JAN 1966	4237	972	45.18	11.28	AUG 1967	0.16	DEC 1965	5.13	MAR 1968	25.5	FEB 1969	16.3	DEC 1971

Month	Relative humidity pct.				Wind						Pct. of possible sunshine	Mean sky cover, tenths, sunrise to sunset	Mean number of days											Average station pressure mb.
								Fastest mile					Sunrise to sunset			Precipitation .01 inch or more	Snow, Ice pellets 1.0 inch or more	Thunderstorms	Heavy fog, visibility 1/4 mile or less	Temperatures °F				Elev.
	Hour 01	Hour 07	Hour 13	Hour 19	Mean speed m.p.h.	Prevailing direction	Speed m.p.h.	Direction	Year				Clear	Partly cloudy	Cloudy					Max. 90° and above	Max. (b) 32° and below	Min. 32° and below	Min. 0° and below	2170 feet m.s.l.
	(Local time)																							
(a)	14	14	14	14	14		14		14		14	14	14	14	14	14	14	14	14	14	14	14	14	6
J	81	86	61	70	9.7		40	34	1975		56	6.1	10	7	14	11	1	1	4	0	4	24	1	941.4
F	77	82	55	67	9.9		60	34	1972		63	5.6	10	6	12	9	1	1	3	0	2	22	*	940.6
M	80	85	53	61	9.6		46	35	1969		65	6.0	9	8	14	12	1	3	2	0	*	14	0	940.4
A	79	86	50	56	9.0		44	22	1970		69	5.6	10	9	11	9	0	3	3	0	0	*	0	941.2
M	90	92	58	67	7.2		40	34	1971		62	6.2	8	9	14	12	0	7	6	*	0	*	0	940.2
J	94	95	60	71	6.2		40	36	1977		66	6.2	6	12	12	12	0	8	8	2	0	0	0	942.4
J	96	96	64	75	5.9		43	35	1966		64	6.4	4	14	13	13	0	10	11	3	0	0	0	943.3
A	97	98	64	70	5.5		40	34	1973		55	6.4	5	13	13	13	0	10	16	1	0	0	0	944.7
S	97	98	65	83	5.7		25	34	1976		61	6.4	6	11	13	10	0	4	13	*	0	*	0	943.4
O	92	95	58	76	7.0		35	33	1972		63	5.0	13	8	10	6	0	1	8	0	0	5	0	944.0
N	86	89	57	71	8.4		40	32	1974		61	5.4	11	7	12	9	*	1	4	0	*	14	0	943.2
D	83	86	60	72	9.0		44	34	1965		57	5.9	11	6	14	10	1	1	5	0	1	21	0	941.3
YR	88	91	59	70	7.7		60	34	FEB 1972		61	5.9	103	110	152	126	5	49	84	6	7	104	1	942.2

eans and extremes above are from existing and comparable exposures. Annual extremes have been exceeded at ther sites in the locality as follows: Highest temperature 99 in July 1936; maximum monthly precipitation 13.75 1 August 1940; minimum monthly precipitation T in October 1963; maximum precipitation in 24 hours 7.92 in October 918; maximum monthly snowfall 28.9 in March 1960.

(a) Length of record, years, through the current year unless otherwise noted, based on January data.
(b) 70° and above at Alaskan stations.
* Less than one half.
T Trace.

NORMALS - Based on record for the 1941-1970 period.
DATE OF AN EXTREME - The most recent in cases of multiple occurrence.
PREVAILING WIND DIRECTION - Record through 1963.
WIND DIRECTION - Numerals indicate tens of degrees clockwise from true north. 00 indicates calm.
FASTEST MILE WIND - Speed is fastest observed 1-minute value when the direction is in tens of degrees.

ASHEVILLE, NC

Average Temperature

Year	Jan	Feb	Mar	Apr	May	June	July	Aug	Sept	Oct	Nov	Dec	Annual
1939	40.2	44.4	49.1	54.1	63.9	74.6	74.6	70.4	69.9	59.6	44.6	40.0	57.3
1940	26.4	36.8	43.1	55.7	62.2	71.6	72.8	72.3	65.2	57.2	46.4	43.6	54.5
1941	38.8	33.8	40.7	55.4	65.6	71.8	74.8	75.1	70.4	63.0	46.9	42.7	56.8
1942	37.4	33.3	38.5	55.5	63.9	73.0	74.6	71.8	67.0	57.5	48.4	38.5	55.9
1943	41.4	40.0	44.6	53.7	65.8	73.0	75.2	75.0	64.1	56.4	44.7	39.2	56.1
1944	39.0	43.4	46.4	56.8	66.8	78.0	72.6	72.6	68.2	56.4	47.9	35.9	56.2
1945	37.0	42.3	57.0	55.4	60.5	71.0	73.9	72.8	69.6	55.5	47.0	34.8	56.6
1946	39.4	41.6	54.0	55.0	62.5	70.3	73.8	74.9	66.2	58.4	42.6	42.6	57.5
1947	43.4	30.9	38.0	58.8	63.2	70.1	70.6	74.9	68.4	61.2	45.1	41.1	57.5
1948	32.4	44.0	50.0	58.2	63.8	71.0	70.2	72.4	68.4	61.6	42.1	42.1	57.0
1949	47.1	50.0	47.0	56.4	67.0	73.7	74.0	72.4	64.4	61.6	44.5	43.2	57.9
1950	51.6	44.0	43.8	52.9	67.1	71.3	72.3	74.8	66.4	61.2	42.1	34.8	56.6
1951	38.7	41.8	47.4	54.2	63.1	71.1	74.5	75.2	68.3	59.6	41.3	41.1	56.3
1952	44.3	43.6	46.0	54.4	65.0	76.8	72.6	72.7	66.2	55.4	46.1	39.2	57.1
1953	42.3	43.1	49.2	58.0	68.0	73.7	74.0	73.2	64.4	61.6	43.2	38.9	57.3
1954	40.4	40.8	47.2	61.2	63.0	71.2	74.5	74.5	70.2	57.4	43.2	37.1	56.7
1955	36.8	40.8	40.1	50.5	60.0	65.7	74.8	74.8	68.9	56.4	42.1	37.5	56.2
1956	34.4	44.7	47.2	54.0	65.7	70.0	73.6	73.5	69.0	59.6	45.7	57.8	55.8
1957	39.4	46.4	45.5	55.0	65.8	71.2	72.3	72.3	69.0	52.0	46.4	41.2	57.1
1958	32.2	29.7	41.0	55.5	71.2	72.0	73.4	67.6	50.1	37.0	40.7	56.5
1959	36.5	42.1	44.6	56.0	64.4	69.9	74.4	74.4	67.6	59.9	45.1	40.7	56.7
1960	39.0	36.6	33.5	58.2	61.1	71.1	73.4	74.1	68.9	58.9	47.4	34.7	54.7
1961	33.5	44.1	50.1	50.4	68.6	72.5	72.0	72.0	68.4	58.3	50.4	39.7	55.5
1962	37.4	45.8	50.1	60.4	69.2	72.3	72.0	66.2	56.0	34.4	41.2	55.7
1963	34.4	34.2	51.0	57.5	63.6	71.4	71.4	66.2	53.0	47.5	31.6	54.8
#1965	37.1	35.1	40.4	57.4	65.8	66.8	72.2	71.1	66.0	58.9	46.4	40.3	54.8
1966	30.1	36.2	43.5	57.0	66.1	68.9	69.6	69.6	62.9	51.7	45.0	37.6	52.2
1967	38.7	35.0	49.8	57.6	60.8	68.5	68.5	60.2	51.7	42.7	41.8	53.6
1968	34.3	32.4	49.2	57.0	69.5	74.1	74.1	64.1	50.7	46.0	36.5	53.0
1969	36.7	37.8	41.3	56.7	69.5	75.4	70.7	65.8	59.0	44.0	36.5	55.0
1970	30.9	39.1	44.8	63.7	70.1	73.1	70.9	70.7	59.0	46.0	42.8	56.2
1971	36.5	39.5	43.1	55.2	72.4	72.5	72.5	69.5	61.8	45.5	47.7	56.0
1972	42.1	38.5	51.2	60.2	70.5	72.3	70.0	59.0	55.6	45.2	45.7	55.7
1973	48.5	40.5	52.8	63.7	61.7	74.2	72.9	70.2	58.8	49.3	39.3	56.5
1974	41.7	42.5	54.1	60.0	68.8	72.9	65.2	57.3	48.2	40.3	56.1
1976	33.6	45.3	50.6	54.9	68.1	70.2	70.0	63.1	51.5	41.2	36.2	53.8
1977	24.8	37.4	37.4	58.2	68.7	73.0	69.1	54.3	49.3	36.8	55.3
1978	29.3	33.4	45.9	56.8	71.1	74.1	70.0	55.7	55.7	51.8	41.0	55.4
RECORD MEAN	35.8	38.1	46.6	55.6	62.5	68.1	72.8	72.1	66.6	55.7	46.3	40.1	55.1
RECORD MAX	46.6	49.7	59.0	62.0	69.0	80.6	82.5	77.2	70.0	58.2	50.9	66.7	
RECORD MIN	25.0	26.4	34.4	42.2	57.5	61.7	55.9	43.3	34.4	29.2		

Heating Degree Days

Season	July	Aug	Sept	Oct	Nov	Dec	Jan	Feb	Mar	Apr	May	June	Total
1958-59	0	0	41	292	449	860	877	635	624	249	58	3	4085
1959-60	0	0	21	204	591	747	800	818	969	226	181	2	4359
1960-61	0	2	32	194	522	931	971	582	453	444	169	18	4316
1961-62	2	0	49	295	433	778	851	531	664	371	27	1	4002
1962-63	0	4	91	224	565	941	943	857	572	241	98	6	4392
1963-64	4	0	51	164	513	826	1038	873	572	251	59	8	4359
#1964-65	0	20	40	372	399	679	863	751	691	232	23	27	4103
1965-66	0	1	39	344	550	759	1075	800	660	383	149	42	4808
1966-67	1	7	87	405	593	838	810	834	465	226	185	51	4496
1967-68	2	0	158	251	660	713	947	939	566	306	150	5	4806
1968-69	0	206	42	251	563	605	873	755	729	246	70	7	4449
1969-70	0	8	59	280	623	875	1050	720	557	236	86	3	4497
1970-71	0	0	29	194	565	682	875	707	569	290	137	0	4151
1971-72	0	0	8	149	576	530	704	790	569	294	116	35	3749
1972-73	3	3	8	304	578	605	846	737	374	362	158	0	3975
1973-74	0	0	7	205	473	772	516	680	423	299	83	24	3482
1974-75	0	0	65	316	519	760	760	624	619	331	64	7	4002
1975-76	0	8	77	237	498	812	966	566	439	296	168	33	4087
1976-77	2	3	83	341	706	884	1239	768	437	198	66	25	4822
1977-78	0	0	34	466	466	768	1101	878	586	241	139	0	4624
1978-79	0	0	12	283	390	741							

Cooling Degree Days

Year	Jan	Feb	Mar	Apr	May	June	July	Aug	Sept	Oct	Nov	Dec	Total
1969	0	0	0	4	55	252	343	196	92	15	0	0	997
1970	0	0	0	22	52	159	296	259	206	17	0	0	1011
1971	0	0	0	3	25	232	238	231	149	37	8	0	923
1972	0	0	0	24	6	84	236	237	134	0	1	0	722
1973	0	0	0	3	16	190	236	288	163	9	0	0	969
1974	0	0	0	1	65	82	254	234	92	1	0	0	731
1975	0	0	0	0	82	124	237	252	89	0	0	0	795
1976	0	0	0	0	5	135	198	170	35	2	0	0	545
1977	0	0	0	2	59	173	340	279	146	7	1	0	1007
1978	0	0	0	2	53	188	266	292	108	4	0	0	973

# Indicates a station move or relocation of instruments. See Station Location table.

Record mean values above are means through the current year for the period beginning in 1965. Data are from City Office locations through 1964 and from Airport locations beginning January 1965.

Precipitation

Year	Jan	Feb	Mar	Apr	May	June	July	Aug	Sept	Oct	Nov	Dec	Annual
1939	3.94	5.77	2.56	2.38	2.78	4.21	3.79	5.14	1.61	0.82	0.77	2.08	35.80
1940	2.13	2.01	2.85	3.26	1.99	3.10	4.03	13.75	0.35	1.12	1.36	2.79	39.34
1941	1.13	0.05	3.18	1.80	1.51	3.67	9.61	2.46	1.35	1.28	0.77	2.08	30.32
1942	2.18	3.49	4.69	1.08	4.63	8.28	3.95	3.89	5.39	1.72	0.51	5.43	39.03
1943	3.43	2.12	4.00	1.08	3.96	6.81	2.07	2.17	2.05	0.59	1.59	1.62	39.51
1944	2.52	6.46	5.30	2.73	2.85	1.97	6.24	2.76	3.42	2.06	1.95	2.27	40.53
1945	1.76	4.22	3.55	4.87	2.87	5.04	3.04	3.82	4.47	2.95	2.96	4.83	45.09
1946	4.40	4.29	4.88	3.09	3.87	1.08	6.49	1.78	1.31	5.09	1.21	1.86	39.92
1947	6.04	2.86	2.22	2.42	1.93	3.50	2.56	4.27	1.85	3.93	3.15	2.92	38.17
1948	2.05	3.24	2.11	3.11	2.90	6.52	6.74	4.78	1.60	3.93	1.45	2.92	39.71
1949	2.06	3.14	3.41	1.43	3.03	4.19	4.10	2.65	1.53	1.81	1.45	4.11	41.80
1950	3.14	2.06	3.91	1.78	4.03	3.06	3.06	3.71	2.25	1.84	1.03	4.11	33.90
1951	1.07	1.80	5.22	2.62	0.59	7.03	2.75	1.50	3.55	1.09	3.20	4.79	35.21
1952	3.09	2.40	7.15	3.72	0.94	3.18	3.18	5.53	2.28	2.23	2.28	2.28	32.81
1953	4.22	4.49	2.10	2.79	3.53	2.40	1.91	2.43	3.04	0.46	1.24	2.67	31.81
1954	6.31	3.04	5.11	1.81	2.78	3.08	2.44	3.10	1.22	2.98	1.45	2.58	37.33
1955	1.11	3.09	4.14	1.55	4.86	2.97	3.06	3.71	0.98	1.39	1.95	0.93	31.70
1956	1.02	4.87	3.57	4.33	2.21	4.44	2.54	1.38	7.11	1.34	2.67	2.96	38.38
1957	4.89	3.03	4.76	6.76	1.03	6.20	3.24	0.98	4.26	1.18	6.22	3.93	42.38
1958	2.89	3.03	7.66	4.04	1.02	2.71	2.93	3.83	1.94	1.88	1.88	2.44	40.02
1959	2.96	1.51	3.37	4.70	7.33	0.80	2.85	3.41	8.33	5.06	1.01	2.88	36.67
1960	2.79	4.19	3.97	3.55	2.11	4.12	4.47	7.24	0.98	1.00	0.68	0.16	37.60
1961	1.45	5.18	3.19	2.98	3.04	4.44	2.54	8.13	1.07	2.36	4.85	6.09	45.32
1962	4.46	3.58	4.13	3.25	2.83	6.20	3.24	3.47	2.40	2.40	2.40	1.66	40.02
1963	1.73	4.13	7.66	4.13	2.53	2.71	2.93	3.83	3.64	1.83	4.42	2.44	36.07
# 1964	2.83	3.58	5.13	5.21	0.94	0.80	8.88	8.88	5.37	8.46	2.51	2.88	49.88
1965	2.16	4.60	5.10	4.21	3.33	4.12	4.47	4.03	4.09	2.92	1.30	0.16	39.50
1966	3.37	6.56	2.59	5.47	4.73	2.45	3.24	7.73	4.55	5.37	3.32	2.36	51.75
1967	2.93	2.20	2.61	2.37	4.95	5.06	6.58	11.28	2.53	4.44	2.54	2.13	51.11
1968	2.64	2.65	0.65	2.37	2.92	3.30	7.53	3.31	2.64	2.03	2.98	3.10	44.78
1969	2.64	5.08	4.01	3.53	3.32	3.82	7.53	6.47	3.04	1.91	1.91	4.63	48.61
1970	1.75	2.42	2.62	2.96	1.72	2.72	5.02	2.46	1.17	5.55	1.83	2.72	32.94
1971	2.53	4.95	3.48	2.06	3.54	5.00	5.47	3.03	3.80	7.05	2.84	4.32	48.05
1972	3.57	2.19	2.19	1.49	6.03	4.66	4.66	5.29	5.29	4.44	4.42	3.89	48.02
1973	4.26	4.23	3.18	5.71	8.83	3.87	6.93	4.57	3.12	2.41	3.57	8.38	64.91
1974	3.64	4.24	4.69	5.86	5.56	3.73	3.31	7.34	3.12	3.83	2.84	2.88	48.44
1975	3.86	4.36	9.86	0.61	8.17	2.29	3.31	3.03	7.53	3.94	4.89	4.44	46.92
1976	3.51	2.20	4.94	0.25	8.67	5.51	5.47	4.23	3.50	5.59	1.58	4.05	47.23
1977	2.09	1.02	7.29	4.05	3.96	5.11	1.03	3.68	9.12	3.70	6.88	2.43	50.45
1978	7.47	0.44	5.22	2.97	4.65	2.29	0.63	6.91	2.57	0.30	2.49	4.32	40.26
RECORD MEAN	3.26	3.22	4.99	2.87	5.20	4.06	4.54	5.04	4.12	3.63	3.20	3.82	48.15

Snowfall

Season	July	Aug	Sept	Oct	Nov	Dec	Jan	Feb	Mar	Apr	May	June	Total
1939-40	0.0	0.0	0.0	0.0	T	4.4	7.7	3.0	3.5	0.2	0.0	0.0	18.8
1940-41	0.0	0.0	0.0	0.0	T	T	T	1.1	4.4	0.0	0.0	0.0	5.5
1941-42	0.0	0.0	0.0	0.0	T	0.4	3.4	2.2	16.0	0.8	0.0	0.0	23.0
1942-43	0.0	0.0	0.0	0.0	T	4.4	T	2.1	1.1	0.6	0.0	0.0	15.7
1943-44	0.0	0.0	0.0	0.0	0.6	6.4	T	1.0	0.0	0.0	0.0	0.0	8.0
1944-45	0.0	0.0	0.0	0.0	T	11.05	4.2	11.0	T	T	0.0	0.0	15.2
1945-46	0.0	0.0	0.0	0.0	0.0	10.5	7.7	8.4	8.5	0.0	0.0	0.0	20.0
1946-47	0.0	0.0	0.0	0.0	0.0	2.4	T	0.1	1.0	0.0	0.0	0.0	20.5
1947-48	0.0	0.0	0.0	0.0	0.8	0.2	3.2	T	T	0.7	0.0	0.0	3.4
1948-49	0.0	0.0	0.0	0.0	0.0	0.2	0.0	0.1	0.1	T	0.0	0.0	1.2
1949-50	0.0	0.0	0.0	0.0	3.1	1.1	0.4	3.3	1.2	T	0.0	0.0	5.7
1950-51	0.0	0.0	0.0	0.0	1.0	1.1	2.8	8.9	T	T	0.0	0.0	6.8
1951-52	0.0	0.0	0.0	0.0	0.0	1.2	3.6	3.1	1.2	T	0.0	0.0	13.5
1952-53	0.0	0.0	0.0	0.0	0.8	1.5	0.0	3.5	1.8	T	0.0	0.0	9.7
1953-54	0.0	0.0	0.0	T	0.2	2.8	0.0	0.1	T	0.2	0+	0.0	9.5
1954-55	0.0	0.0	0.0	0.0	0.0	2.6	2.0	0.1	T	0.0	0.0	0.0	—
1955-56	0.0	0.0	0.0	0.0	1.0	0.6	3.4	0.1	1.1	2.0	0.0	0.0	8.3
1956-57	0.0	0.0	0.0	T	0.3	0.25	0.8	12.8	2.5	0+	0.0	0.0	3.6
1957-58	0.0	0.0	0.0	T	T	1.3	T	T	1.9	T	0+	0.0	7.4
1958-59	0.0	0.0	0.0	0.0	T	1.0	2.0	8.5	26.9	0.2	0.0	0.0	41.1
1959-60	0.0	0.0	0.0	0.0	T	1.2	0.0	T	T	T	0.0	0.0	40.6
1960-61	0.0	0.0	0.0	T	T	0.8	0.8	3.0	T	T	0.0	0.0	4.0
1961-62	0.0	0.0	0.0	0+	T	1.2	13.3	4.5	8.3	T	0.0	0.0	22.8
1962-63	0.0	0.0	0.0	0.0	0.3	4.2	1.7	12.9	0.1	0.0	0.0	0.0	9.0
1963-64	0.0	0.0	0.0	0.0	1.2	8.9	5.5	4.3	5.0	0.0	0.0	0.0	25.8
# 1964-65	0.0	0.0	0.0	0.0	T	T	T	T	T	T	0.0	0.0	14.8
1965-66	0.0	0.0	0.0	0.0	1.3	2.1	17.6	6.2	0.2	T	0.0	0.0	24.0
1966-67	0.0	0.0	0.0	0.0	1.5	0.1	6.9	4.2	T	0+	0.0	0.0	17.8
1967-68	0.0	0.0	0.0	0.0	9.0	T	7.2	0.2	0.1	0.0	0.0	0.0	15.2
1968-69	0.0	0.0	0.0	0.0	T	10.9	6.0	25.1	13.0	0.0	0.0	0.0	48.2
1969-70	0.0	0.0	0.0	0.0	0.0	T	T	1.1	0.5	0.0	0.0	0.0	17.5
1970-71	0.0	0.0	0.0	0.0	T	6.1	0.1	0.1	8.9	0.2	0.0	0.0	15.4
1971-72	0.0	0.0	0.0	0.0	0.6	16.3	7.1	7.5	7.4	0+	0.0	0.0	31.7
1972-73	0.0	0.0	0.0	0.0	0.0	3.0	T	0.1	1.7	T	0.0	0.0	9.2
1973-74	0.0	0.0	0.0	0.0	3.1	3.0	0.4	4.3	1.7	T	0.0	0.0	4.4
1974-75	0.0	0.0	0.0	0.0	T	T	T	T	T	T	0.0	0.0	14.5
1975-76	0.0	0.0	0.0	0+	5.0	0.4	1.0	3.5	T	0.0	0.0	0.0	10.5
1976-77	0.0	0.0	0.0	0.7	0.1	0.1	6.7	5.1	0.3	T	0.0	0.0	21.8
1977-78	0.0	0.0	0.0	0.0	T	T	9.7	T	5.3	0+	0.0	0.0	—
1978-79	0.0	0.0	0.0	0.0	0.0	T							
RECORD MEAN	0.0	0.0	T	T	1.5	3.2	4.8	5.0	3.3	T	0.0	0.0	17.8

# Indicates a station move or relocation of instruments. See Station Location table.

Record mean values above are means through the current year for the period beginning in 1965. Data are from City Office locations through 1964 and from Airport locations beginning January 1965.

Following are two samples of the Monthly Summaries issued by the National Climatic Center. These are for Phoenix for the months of January and July, 1979.

LOCAL CLIMATOLOGICAL DATA

JANUARY 1979
PHOENIX. ARIZONA
NAT WEATHER SERVICE FCST OFC
SKY HARBOR INTL AIRPORT

MONTHLY SUMMARY

LATITUDE 33° 26' N   LONGITUDE 112° 01' W   ELEVATION (GROUND)   1110 FT.   STANDARD TIME USED: MOUNTAIN   WBAN #23183

DATE	TEMPERATURE °F MAXIMUM	MINIMUM	AVERAGE	DEPARTURE FROM NORMAL	AVERAGE DEW POINT	DEGREE DAYS BASE 65° HEATING (SEASON BEGINS WITH JULY)	COOLING (SEASON BEGINS WITH JAN.)	WEATHER TYPES ON DATES OF OCCURRENCE 1 FOG 2 HEAVY FOG 3 THUNDERSTORM 4 ICE PELLETS 5 HAIL 6 GLAZE 7 DUSTSTORM 8 SMOKE,HAZE 9 BLOWING SNOW	SNOW,ICE PELLETS OR ICE ON GROUND AT 05AM IN.	PRECIPITATION WATER EQUIVALENT IN	SNOW,ICE PELLETS IN.	AVG. STATION PRES. SURE IN. ELEV. 1107 FEET M.S.L.	WIND RESULTANT DIR.	RESULTANT SPEED M.P.H.	AVERAGE SPEED M.P.H.	FASTEST MILE SPEED M.P.H.	DIRECTION	SUNSHINE MINUTES	PERCENT OF POSSIBLE	SKY COVER TENTHS SUNRISE TO SUNSET	MIDNIGHT TO MIDNIGHT
1	2	3	4	5	6	7A	7B	8	9	10	11	12	13	14	15	16	17	18	19	20	21
1	57	34	46	-5	19	19	0		0	0	0	29.22	02	6.4	9.6	29	N/	599	100	0	0
2	56	30	43	-8	16	22	0		0	0	0	29.20	33	2.0	7.5	20	E/	522	87	8	7
3	58	41	50	-1	30	15	0		0	0	0	28.99	14	1.7	5.6	15	SE/	165	28	10	9
4	70*	37	54	3	36	11	0		0	0	0	29.01	14	3.7	6.2	13	E/	540	90	4	3
5	59	46	53	2	44	12	0		0	.07	0	28.87	10	4.5	6.9	18	SE/	10	2	10	9
6	63	46	55	4	48	10	0		0	0	0	28.84	18	2.2	4.9	13	E/	420	70	5	7
7	60	48	54	3	48	11	0		0	0	0	28.97	24	3.6	5.3	12	W/	264	44	10	8
8	65	42	54	3	44	11	0	8	0	0	0	29.02	17	2.0	4.3	10	W/	529	88	7	5
9	54	44	49	-2	45	16	0	1 8	0	.04	0	28.92	26	1.4	6.0	17	SW/	1	0	10	8
10	57	41	49	-2	45	16	0	2 8	0	0	0	29.03	18	2.8	5.6	12	SW/	284	47	7	6
11	63	40	52	1	44	13	0	2 8	0	0	0	28.94	10	3.6	5.3	12	E/	337	56	7	7
12	66	47	57	6	46	8	0	1 8	0	0	0	28.77	17	2.6	7.6	25	N/	359	59	8	8
13	65	39	52	1	37	13	0		0	0	0	28.92	15	2.9	5.5	14	E/	543	89	6	3
14	63	41	52	1	34	13	0		0	T	0	28.87	10	1.8	6.5	18	W/	153	25	10	10
15	63	49	56	5	45	9	0		0	T	0	28.80	10	5.3	8.3	22	E/	43	7	10	10
16	58	53	56	5	50	9	0		0	.42	0	28.80	08	6.7	9.1	23	E/	2	0	10	10
17	63	53	58*	7	53	7	0		0	.73	0	28.71	14	.7	6.0	17	E/	91	15	10	10
18	61	48	55	4	50	10	0	3	0	.36	0	28.81	16	5.5	8.5	29	W/	113	18	9	9
19	56	44	50	-1	44	15	0	2	0	T	0	28.90	09	3.2	8.3	23	E/	288	47	8	5
20	62	37	50	-1	39	15	0		0	0	0	29.01	21	1.7	6.0	14	W/	601	97	2	2
21	62	41	52	1	38	13	0		0	0	0	28.82	32	.3	7.1	14	SW/	241	39	10	10
22	62	44	53	2	42	12	0		0	T	0	28.72	25	2.5	7.9	24	W/	598	96	1	3
23	59	37	48	-3	35	17	0		0	0	0	28.83	18	.9	5.5	13	W/	583	94	3	2
24	58	40	49	-2	37	16	0		0	.14	0	28.63	08	4.4	7.6	17	NE/	12	2	10	10
25	55	44	50	-1	43	15	0	1 3	0	.11	0	28.50	20	3.7	8.1	30	W/	28	4	10	10
26	55	40	48	-4	35	17	0		0	0	0	28.82	25	6.3	7.1	23	W/	590	94	3	3
27	53	33	43	-9	28	22	0		0	0	0	28.93	19	2.9	6.0	12	W/	627	100	0	0
28	55	33	44	-8	33	21	0		0	.29	0	28.69	13	3.9	9.1	29	W/	408	65	4	4
29	49	34	42	-10	29	23	0	8	0	0	0	28.85	25	8.7	9.8	24	W/	506	80	3	4
30	50	29*	40*	-12	24	25	0		0	0	0	28.92	11	4.5	7.1	17	NE/	631	100	0	0
31	59	32	46	-7	29	19	0		0	0	0	28.88	13	4.5	7.6	18	E/	279	44	8	7

| SUM 1836 | SUM 1267 | | | | | TOTAL 455 | TOTAL 0 | | | TOTAL 2.16 | TOTAL 0 | 28.88 | 15 | 1.5 | 7.0 FOR THE MONTH: 30 | W/ | TOTAL 10367 | FOR 204 | SUM 187 | SUM |
| AVG. 59.2 | AVG. 40.9 | AVG. 50.1 | DEP. -1.1 | AVG. 38 | DEP. | DEP. | | | PRECIPITATION >.01 INCH 8 | DEP. | | | | DATE: 25 | POSSIBLE 19018 | MONTH 55 | AVG. 6.6 | AVG. 6.0 |

NUMBER OF DAYS
MAXIMUM TEMP. ≥ 90° 0 | < 32° 0 | MINIMUM TEMP. ≤ 32° 3 | ≤ 0° 0

SEASON TO DATE
TOTAL 1009 HEATING | TOTAL 0 COOLING | DEP. | DEP. | -6 PRECIPITATION

NUMBER OF DAYS
PRECIPITATION > 1.0 INCH 0
> .01 INCH 8
SNOW, ICE PELLETS > 1.0 INCH 0
THUNDERSTORMS 2
HEAVY FOG 3
CLEAR 8   PARTLY CLOUDY 7   CLOUDY 16

GREATEST IN 24 HOURS AND DATES
PRECIPITATION 1.08 16-17
SNOW, ICE PELLETS 0

GREATEST DEPTH ON GROUND OF SNOW,
ICE PELLETS OR ICE AND DATE
0

* EXTREME FOR THE MONTH - LAST OCCURRENCE IF MORE THAN ONE.
T TRACE AMOUNT
• ALSO ON AN EARLIER DATE, OR DATES.
HEAVY FOG - VISIBILITY 1/4 MILE OR LESS.
FIGURES FOR WIND DIRECTIONS ARE TENS OF DEGREES CLOCKWISE FROM TRUE NORTH. 00 - CALM.
DATA IN COLS. 6 AND 12-15 ARE BASED ON 7 OR

MORE OBSERVATIONS PER DAY AT 3-HOUR INTERVALS.
FASTEST MILE WIND SPEEDS ARE FASTEST OBSERVED ONE-MINUTE VALUES WHEN DIRECTIONS ARE IN TENS OF DEGREES. THE / WITH THE DIRECTION INDICATES PEAK GUST SPEED.
ANY ERRORS DETECTED WILL BE CORRECTED AND CHANGES IN SUMMARY DATA WILL BE ANNOTATED IN THE ANNUAL SUMMARY

PILOT REPORTED A FUNNEL CLOUD 15 MILES SE OF AIRPORT AT 1730 LST
ON JAN. 25TH.

SUMMARY BY HOURS

HOUR LOCAL TIME	AVERAGES SKY COVER TENTHS	STATION PRESSURE IN.	TEMPERATURE AIR °F	WET BULB °F	DEW PT. °F	RELATIVE HUMIDITY %	WIND SPEED M.P.H.	RESULTANT WIND DIRECTION	SPEED M.P.H.
02	5	28.88	45	42	39	81	6.5	12	2.3
05	6	28.88	43	41	39	86	6.0	16	2.7
08	7	28.90	43	41	38	86	6.2	13	2.5
11	6	28.93	52	45	38	61	7.7	10	3.1
14	7	28.86	57	48	36	49	8.8	17	1.4
17	7	28.84	57	48	37	50	8.1	23	2.8
20	6	28.86	51	45	39	67	6.2	25	1.4
23	5	28.86	47	44	40	77	6.5	12	1.4

LOCAL CLIMATOLOGICAL DATA

1979

NIX. ARIZONA
WEATHER SERVICE FCST OFC
HARBOR INTL AIRPORT

MONTHLY SUMMARY

UDE 33° 26 'N   LONGITUDE 112° 01 'W   ELEVATION (GROUND)   1110 FT.   STANDARD TIME USED: MOUNTAIN   WBAN #23183

	TEMPERATURE °F					DEGREE DAYS BASE 65°		WEATHER TYPES ON DATES OF OCCURRENCE 1 FOG 2 HEAVY FOG 3 THUNDERSTORM 4 ICE PELLETS 5 HAIL 6 GLAZE 7 DUSTSTORM 8 SMOKE. HAZE 9 BLOWING SNOW	SNOW. ICE PELLETS OR ICE ON GROUND AT 05AM IN.	PRECIPITATION		AVG. STATION PRES. SURE IN. . . . ELEV. 1107 M.S.L.	WIND					SUNSHINE		SKY COVER TENTHS		
MAXIMUM	MINIMUM	AVERAGE	DEPARTURE FROM NORMAL	AVERAGE DEW POINT	HEATING (SEASON BEGINS WITH JULY)	COOLING (SEASON BEGINS WITH JAN.)			WATER EQUIVA LENT IN.	SNOW. ICE PELLETS IN.		RESULTANT DIR.	RESULTANT SPEED M.P.H.	AVERAGE SPEED M.P.H.	SPEED M.P.H.	DIRECTION	MINUTES	PERCENT OF POSSIBLE	SUNRISE TO SUNSET	MIDNIGHT TO MIDNIGHT	DATE
2	3	4	5	6	7A	7B	8	9	10	11	12	13	14	15	16	17	18	19	20	21	22
104	84	94	5	54	0	29		0	T	0	28.62	14	8.9	9.6	23	E/	601	70	6	7	1
105	80	93	4	46	0	28		0	0	0	28.63	18	.6	7.8	22	NW/	860	100	2	3	2
106	76	91	1	34	0	26		0	0	0	28.68	17	1.9	10.6	29	W/	788	92	2	2	3
107	73	90	0	33	0	25		0	0	0	28.70	11	4.0	8.5	25	S/	859	100	0	0	4
107	74	91	1	35	0	26		0	0	0	28.70	18	.9	7.3	22	W/	858	100	0	0	5
107	74	91	1	38	0	26		0	0	0	28.73	04	1.7	6.3	17	NW/	857	100	1	0	6
111	73×	92	2	37	0	27		0	0	0	28.73	19	2.1	6.3	16	W/	857	100	0	0	7
111	74	93	2	37	0	28		0	0	0	28.74	26	1.1	6.6	20	W/	856	100	2	1	8
114×	75	95	4	33	0	30		0	0	0	28.68	12	1.3	6.8	21	W/	856	100	0	0	9
113	74	94	3	36	0	29		0	0	0	28.65	26	2.6	8.8	23	W/	854	100	0	0	10
111	76	94	3	37	0	29		0	0	0	28.57	14	.1	7.1	22	W/	853	100	1	1	11
111	77	94	3	40	0	29		0	0	0	28.56	29	1.4	8.1	16	W/	853	100	6	4	12
108	81	95	4	58	0	30		0	0	0	28.64	29	2.0	6.2	20	W/	851	100	0	0	13
108	80	94	2	53	0	29		0	0	0	28.66	28	5.9	6.8	22	NW/	850	100	2	2	14
113	81	97	5	54	0	32		0	0	0	28.63	22	2.4	6.9	15	SW/	752	88	7	7	15
109	86	98	6	57	0	33		0	0	0	28.77	26	1.9	8.2	35	SE/	801	94	4	4	16
108	84	96	4	62	0	31	3	0	.02	0	28.81	33	3.3	7.3	40	NE/	736	87	5	6	17
106	85	96	4	61	0	31		0	T	0	28.71	10	9.4	11.7	30	NE/	686	81	4	5	18
102	81	92	0	65	0	27		0	0	0	28.71	13	6.6	7.8	22	S/	609	72	9	8	19
94	78	86×	-6	68	0	21		0	.02	0	28.74	17	4.4	7.5	25	NE/	377	45	9	9	20
104	80	92	0	63	0	27		0	0	0	28.74	26	2.0	6.8	25	NW/	808	96	1	1	21
106	79	93	1	58	0	28		0	0	0	28.69	25	4.2	7.3	25	W/	772	92	6	4	22
110	78	94	2	50	0	29		0	0	0	28.61	27	5.5	7.2	23	W/	841	100	0	0	23
112	80	96	4	48	0	31		0	0	0	28.58	14	2.9	6.9	18	W/	772	92	5	4	24
111	83	97	5	54	0	32		0	0	0	28.61	30	1.3	8.6	30	W/	838	100	0	0	25
110	83	97	5	59	0	32		0	0	0	28.62	26	6.7	7.2	20	W/	833	100	2	1	26
111	86	99	7	59	0	34		0	0	0	28.59	27	4.2	8.2	17	W/	804	96	0	0	27
113	87	100×	8	59	0	35		0	0	0	28.60	18	1.2	10.1	35	S/	804	96	1	2	28
108	82	95	4	64	0	30	3	0	.30	0	28.68	01	1.7	10.6	47	NE/	698	84	4	5	29
104	78	91	0	67	0	26		0	0	0	28.76	22	3.1	8.9	30	E/	799	96	2	1	30
107	84	96	5	58	0	31		0	0	0	28.75	22	10.9	11.7	25	W/	807	97	0	0	31

	SUM				TOTAL	TOTAL			TOTAL	TOTAL		FOR THE MONTH:			TOTAL	%	SUM	SUM	
3351	2466				0	901			.34	0	28.67	22	1.2	8.1	47	NE/	24390		81	77
AVG.	AVG.	AVG.	DEP.	AVG.	DEP.	DEP.	NUMBER OF DAYS		PRECIPITATION	DEP.		DATE: 29		POSSIBLE MONTH		AVG.	AVG.	
108.1	79.5	93.8	2.6	51	0	89	>.01 INCH	3	>.01 INCH	-0.41				26267	93	2.6	2.5	

NUMBER OF DAYS		SEASON TO DATE TOTAL	TOTAL	SNOW. ICE PELLETS		GREATEST IN 24 HOURS AND DATES		GREATEST DEPTH ON GROUND OF SNOW.
MAXIMUM TEMP.	MINIMUM TEMP.	0	2255	>1.0 INCH	0	PRECIPITATION	SNOW. ICE PELLETS	ICE PELLETS OR ICE AND DATE
>90	<32	<32	<0	DEP.	DEP.	THUNDERSTORMS 2	PRECIPITATION	SNOW. ICE PELLETS
31	0	0	0	0	324	HEAVY FOG 0	.30	29
						CLEAR 20 PARTLY CLOUDY 9 CLOUDY 2		

* EXTREME FOR THE MONTH - LAST OCCURRENCE IF MORE THAN ONE.
T TRACE AMOUNT
+ ALSO ON AN EARLIER DATE. OR DATES.
HEAVY FOG: - VISIBILITY 1/4 MILE OR LESS.
FIGURES FOR WIND DIRECTIONS ARE TENS OF DE-
GREES CLOCKWISE FROM TRUE NORTH. 00 - CALM.
DATA IN COLS. 6 AND 12-15 ARE BASED ON 7 OR

MORE OBSERVATIONS PER DAY AT 3-HOUR INTERVALS.
FASTEST MILE WIND SPEEDS ARE FASTEST OBSERVED
ONE-MINUTE VALUES WHEN DIRECTIONS ARE IN TENS
OF DEGREES. THE / WITH THE DIRECTION INDICATES
PEAK GUST SPEED.
ANY ERRORS DETECTED WILL BE CORRECTED AND
CHANGES IN SUMMARY DATA WILL BE ANNOTATED IN
THE ANNUAL SUMMARY

SUMMARY BY HOURS

	AVERAGES							RESULTANT WIND	
HOUR LOCAL TIME	SKY COVER TENTHS	STATION PRESSURE IN.	TEMPERATURE				RELATIVE HUMIDITY %	WIND SPEED M.P.H.	DIRECTION	SPEED M.P.H.
			AIR °F	WET BULB °F	DEW PT. °F				
02	2	28.67	86	66	54	35	7.8	11	2.9
05	2	28.69	82	65	53	38	7.5	10	5.8
08	3	28.74	88	67	53	33	7.2	11	5.4
11	3	28.73	97	69	52	25	6.8	21	.7
14	2	28.68	104	71	49	18	10.1	26	6.1
17	2	28.61	106	70	47	16	9.4	27	6.8
20	3	28.62	99	69	49	21	8.5	27	4.4
23	2	28.66	91	67	51	28	7.1	24	2.4

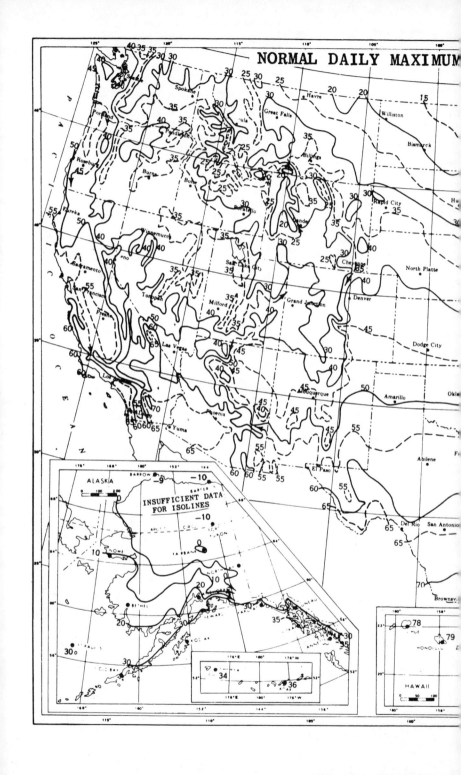

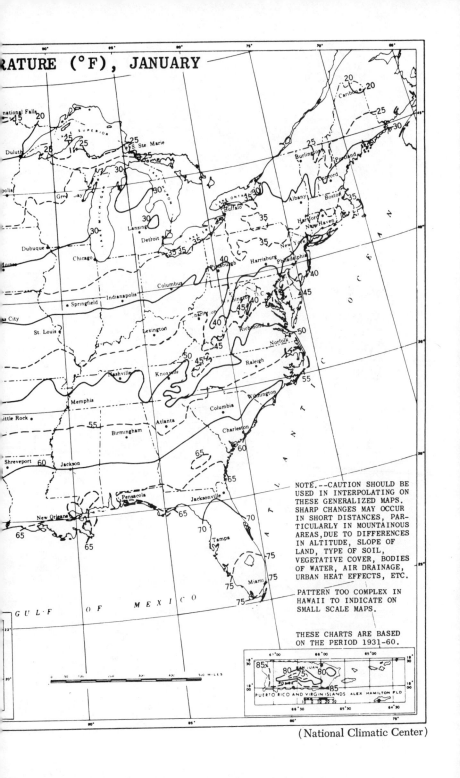

RATURE (°F), JANUARY

NOTE.--CAUTION SHOULD BE
USED IN INTERPOLATING ON
THESE GENERALIZED MAPS.
SHARP CHANGES MAY OCCUR
IN SHORT DISTANCES, PAR-
TICULARLY IN MOUNTAINOUS
AREAS, DUE TO DIFFERENCES
IN ALTITUDE, SLOPE OF
LAND, TYPE OF SOIL,
VEGETATIVE COVER, BODIES
OF WATER, AIR DRAINAGE,
URBAN HEAT EFFECTS, ETC.

PATTERN TOO COMPLEX IN
HAWAII TO INDICATE ON
SMALL SCALE MAPS.

THESE CHARTS ARE BASED
ON THE PERIOD 1931-60.

PUERTO RICO AND VIRGIN ISLANDS   ALEX HAMILTON FLD

(National Climatic Center)

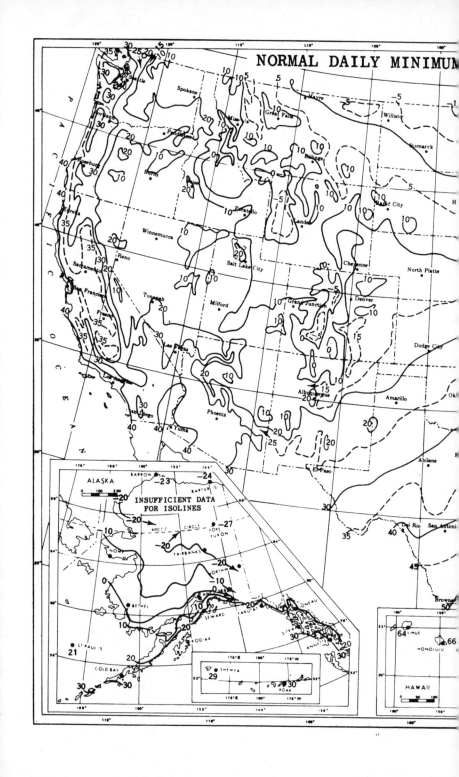

NORMAL DAILY MINIMUM

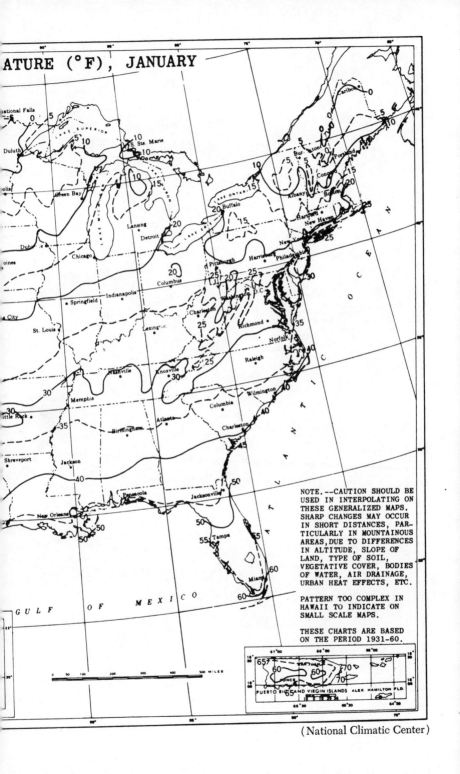

ATURE (°F), JANUARY

NOTE.--CAUTION SHOULD BE
USED IN INTERPOLATING ON
THESE GENERALIZED MAPS.
SHARP CHANGES MAY OCCUR
IN SHORT DISTANCES, PAR-
TICULARLY IN MOUNTAINOUS
AREAS, DUE TO DIFFERENCES
IN ALTITUDE, SLOPE OF
LAND, TYPE OF SOIL,
VEGETATIVE COVER, BODIES
OF WATER, AIR DRAINAGE,
URBAN HEAT EFFECTS, ETC.

PATTERN TOO COMPLEX IN
HAWAII TO INDICATE ON
SMALL SCALE MAPS.

THESE CHARTS ARE BASED
ON THE PERIOD 1931-60.

(National Climatic Center)

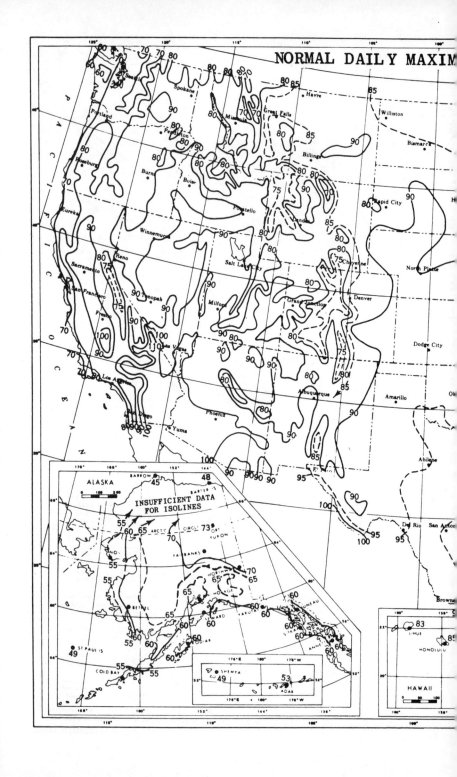

NORMAL DAILY MAXIM

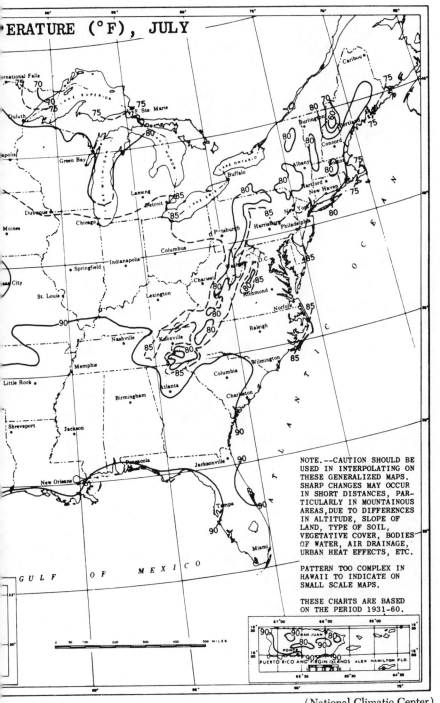

ERATURE (°F), JULY

NOTE.--CAUTION SHOULD BE
USED IN INTERPOLATING ON
THESE GENERALIZED MAPS.
SHARP CHANGES MAY OCCUR
IN SHORT DISTANCES, PAR-
TICULARLY IN MOUNTAINOUS
AREAS, DUE TO DIFFERENCES
IN ALTITUDE, SLOPE OF
LAND, TYPE OF SOIL,
VEGETATIVE COVER, BODIES
OF WATER, AIR DRAINAGE,
URBAN HEAT EFFECTS, ETC.

PATTERN TOO COMPLEX IN
HAWAII TO INDICATE ON
SMALL SCALE MAPS.

THESE CHARTS ARE BASED
ON THE PERIOD 1931-60.

(National Climatic Center)

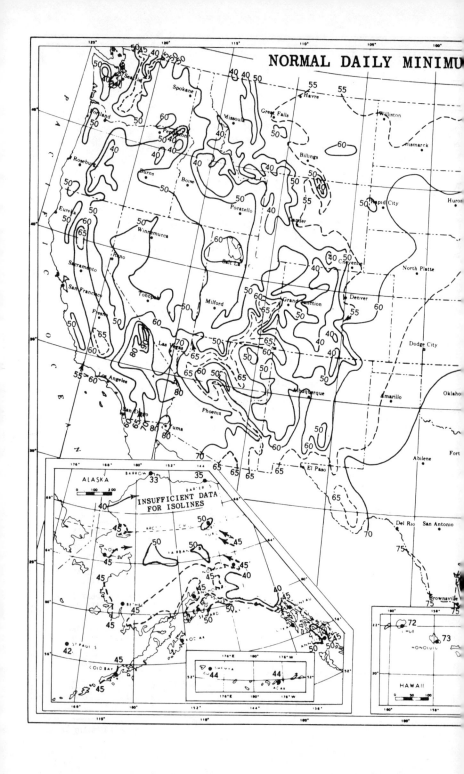

NORMAL DAILY MINIMU

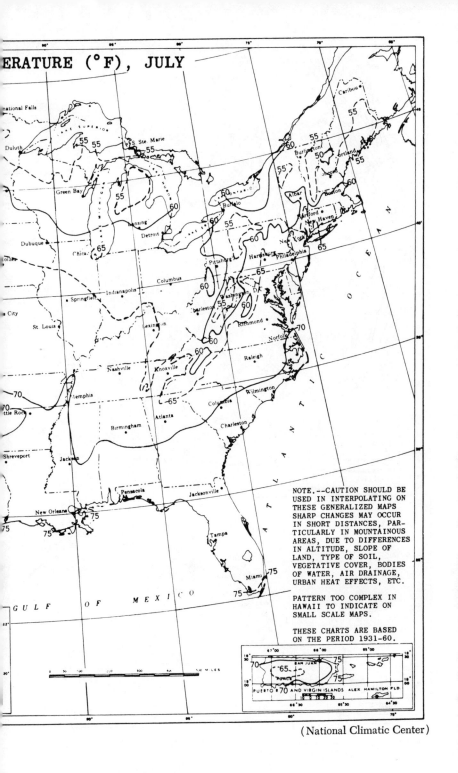

ERATURE (°F), JULY

NOTE.--CAUTION SHOULD BE USED IN INTERPOLATING ON THESE GENERALIZED MAPS SHARP CHANGES MAY OCCUR IN SHORT DISTANCES, PARTICULARLY IN MOUNTAINOUS AREAS, DUE TO DIFFERENCES IN ALTITUDE, SLOPE OF LAND, TYPE OF SOIL, VEGETATIVE COVER, BODIES OF WATER, AIR DRAINAGE, URBAN HEAT EFFECTS, ETC.

PATTERN TOO COMPLEX IN HAWAII TO INDICATE ON SMALL SCALE MAPS.

THESE CHARTS ARE BASED ON THE PERIOD 1931-60.

(National Climatic Center)

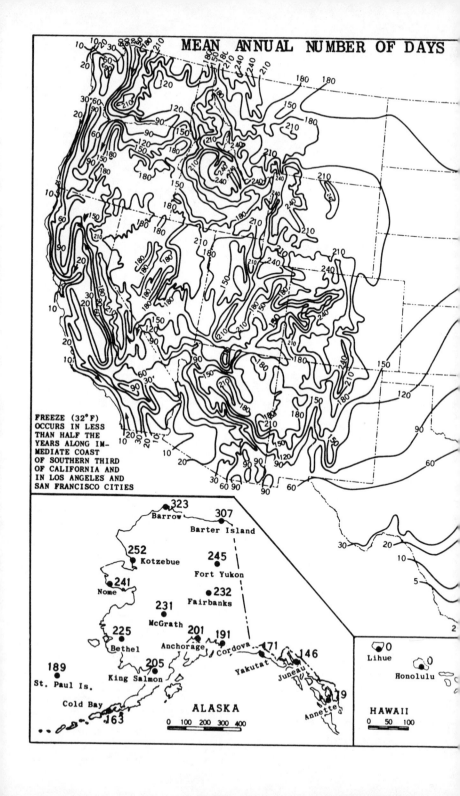

MEAN ANNUAL NUMBER OF DAYS

FREEZE (32°F) OCCURS IN LESS THAN HALF THE YEARS ALONG IMMEDIATE COAST OF SOUTHERN THIRD OF CALIFORNIA AND IN LOS ANGELES AND SAN FRANCISCO CITIES

ALASKA

Barrow **323**
Barter Island **307**
Kotzebue **252**
Fort Yukon **245**
Nome **241**
Fairbanks **232**
McGrath **231**
Anchorage **201**
Cordova **191**
Bethel **225**
Yakutat **171**
Juneau **146**
King Salmon **205**
St. Paul Is. **189**
Cold Bay **163**
Annette **119**

0 100 200 300 400

HAWAII

Lihue **0**
Honolulu **0**

0 50 100

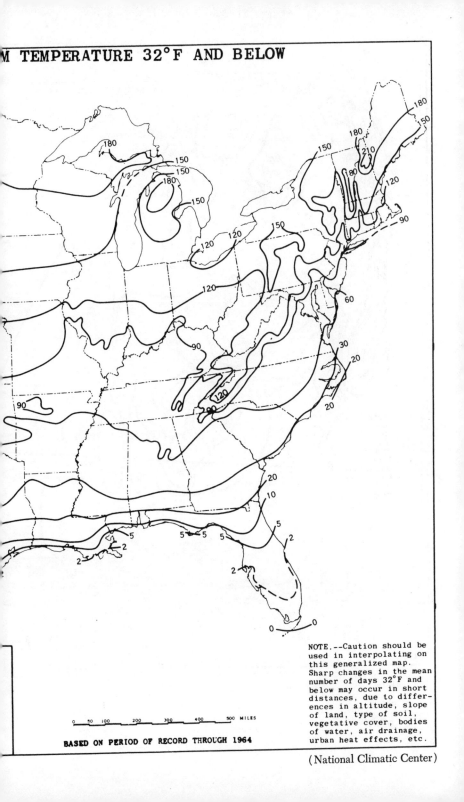

M TEMPERATURE 32°F AND BELOW

NOTE.--Caution should be
used in interpolating on
this generalized map.
Sharp changes in the mean
number of days 32°F and
below may occur in short
distances, due to differ-
ences in altitude, slope
of land, type of soil,
vegetative cover, bodies
of water, air drainage,
urban heat effects, etc.

0   50 100   200   300   400   500 MILES

BASED ON PERIOD OF RECORD THROUGH 1964

(National Climatic Center)

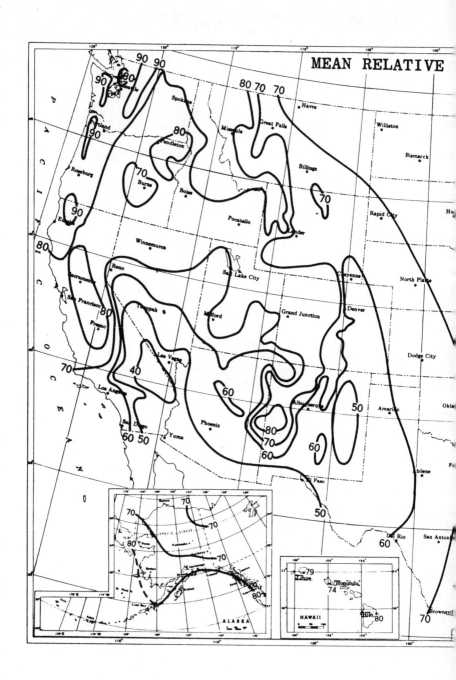

MEAN RELATIVE

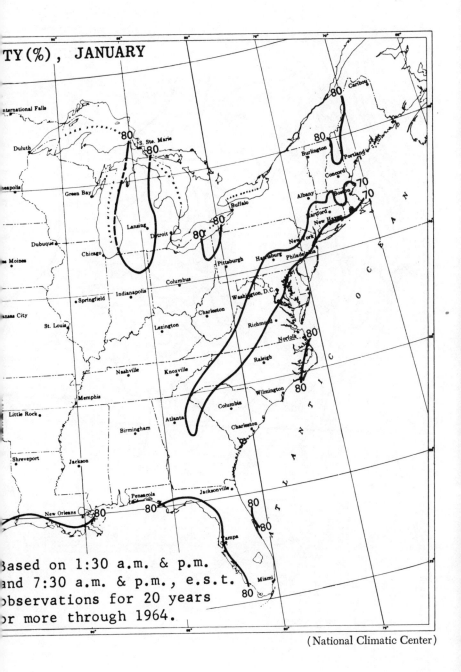

TY(%), JANUARY

Based on 1:30 a.m. & p.m. and 7:30 a.m. & p.m., e.s.t. observations for 20 years or more through 1964.

(National Climatic Center)

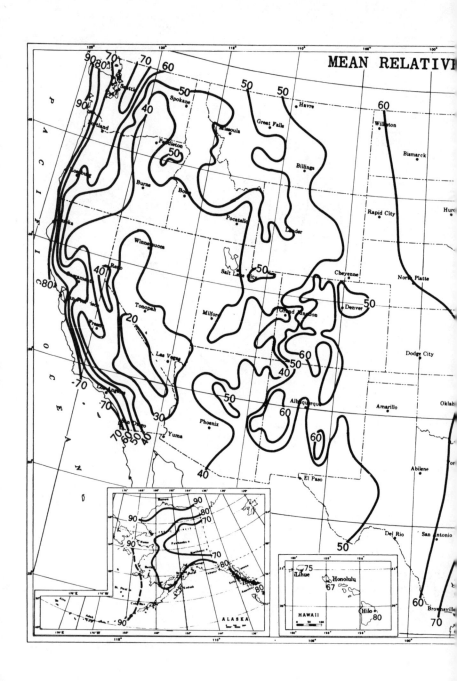

MEAN RELATIVE

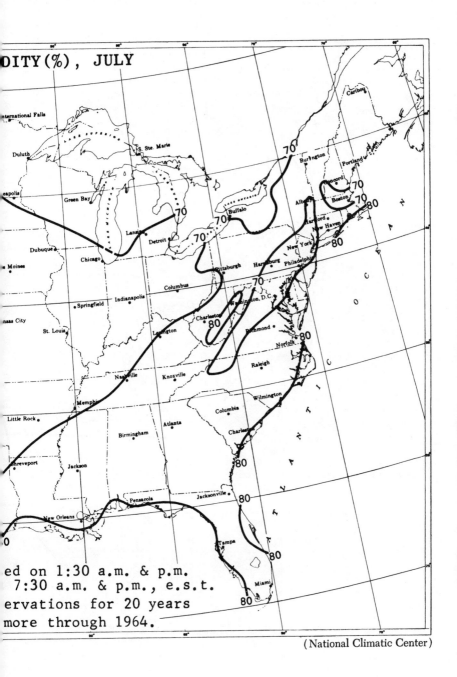

DITY(%), JULY

ed on 1:30 a.m. & p.m.
  7:30 a.m. & p.m., e.s.t.
ervations for 20 years
more through 1964.

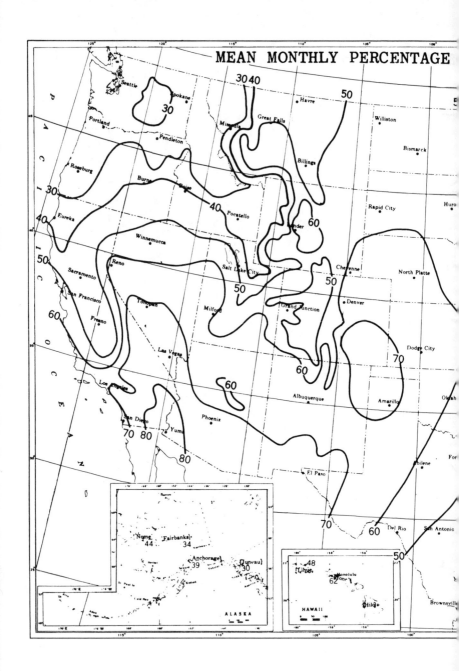

MEAN MONTHLY PERCENTAGE

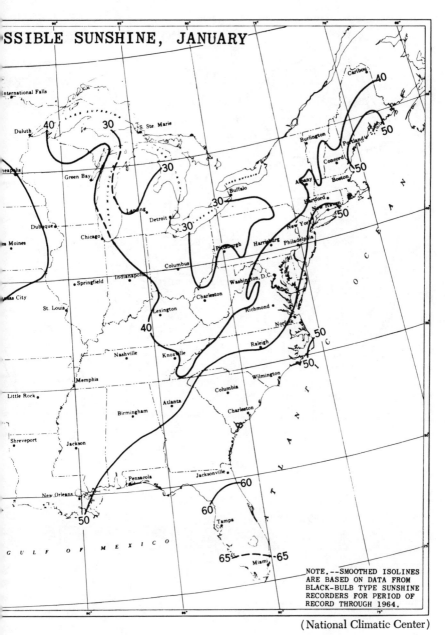

SSIBLE SUNSHINE, JANUARY

NOTE.--SMOOTHED ISOLINES
ARE BASED ON DATA FROM
BLACK-BULB TYPE SUNSHINE
RECORDERS FOR PERIOD OF
RECORD THROUGH 1964.

(National Climatic Center)

Appendix 199

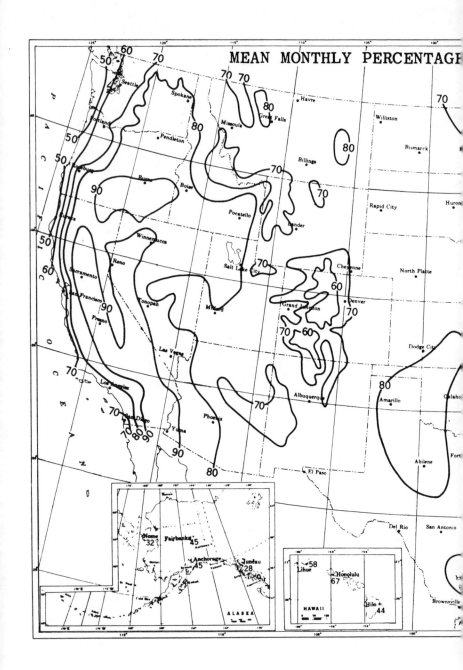

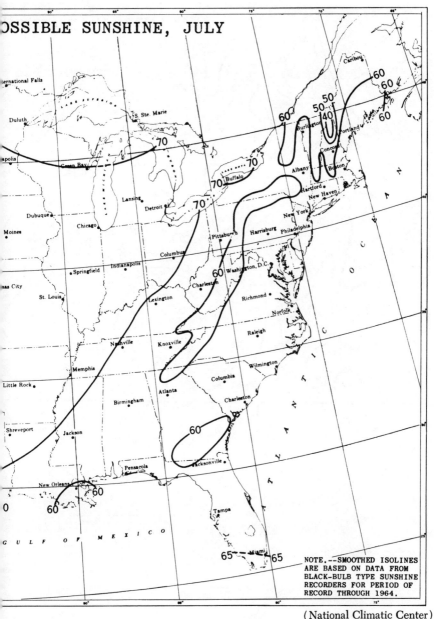

OSSIBLE SUNSHINE, JULY

NOTE.--SMOOTHED ISOLINES
ARE BASED ON DATA FROM
BLACK-BULB TYPE SUNSHINE
RECORDERS FOR PERIOD OF
RECORD THROUGH 1964.

(National Climatic Center)

Appendix   201

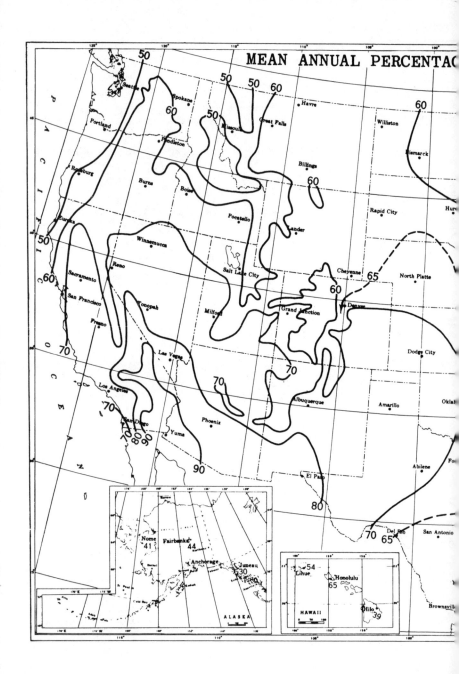

MEAN ANNUAL PERCENTA

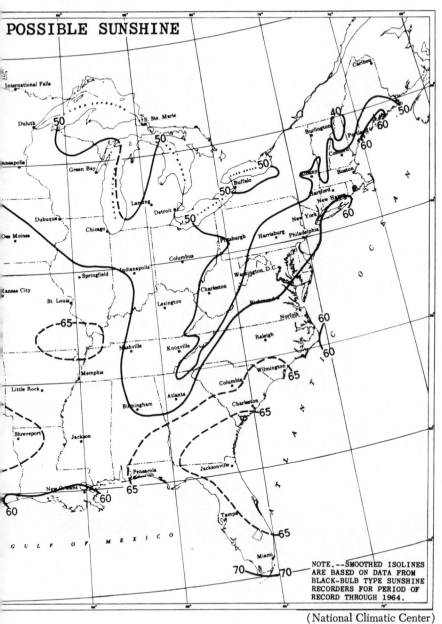

POSSIBLE SUNSHINE

NOTE.--SMOOTHED ISOLINES
ARE BASED ON DATA FROM
BLACK-BULB TYPE SUNSHINE
RECORDERS FOR PERIOD OF
RECORD THROUGH 1964.

(National Climatic Center)

Appendix 203